Systems-Centered Training

This illustrated book shows how "thinking" systems offer new ways of seeing people which can help us see and do things differently. The authors describe how a theory of living human systems was developed and even recently revised. This major revision led to a theory of the person-as-a-system and its role-systems map that helps us see which system in us and in others is running the show.

The authors illustrate how life force energy fuels the hierarchy of living human systems and how theory and practice with role-systems can be useful in everyday life. They begin with describing how we can use the new illustrations as a map to locate the contexts of our roles. Using this map helps us to identify the role-systems and explore the territory of ourselves and our groups in new ways that deepen our understanding of roles and role locks.

This book illustrates systems-centered therapy and training (SCT) theory by offering a practical theory to guide group psychotherapists, leaders and consultants in working with group dynamics.

Yvonne M. Agazarian, Ed.D., developed a theory of living human systems and SCT. She loved theorizing and authored six books and many articles about SCT.

Susan P. Gantt, Ph.D., taught group psychotherapy for Emory University School of Medicine, chairs the Systems-Centered Training and Research Institute (SCTRI) and leads ongoing SCT training groups in Atlanta, San Francisco and the Netherlands. She has published widely in SCT.

Frances B. Carter, MSW, is a founding member of SCTRI, co-directs the SCTRI Training and Resource Center and leads SCT training in the US and Europe. She brings her early background as an artist to all her work.

Systems-Centered Training

An Illustrated Guide for Applying a
Theory of Living Human Systems

Yvonne M. Agazarian
Susan P. Gantt
Frances B. Carter

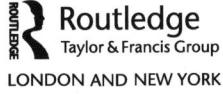
Routledge
Taylor & Francis Group

LONDON AND NEW YORK

First published 2021
by Routledge
2 Park Square, Milton Park, Abingdon, Oxon OX14 4RN

and by Routledge
52 Vanderbilt Avenue, New York, NY 10017

Routledge is an imprint of the Taylor & Francis Group, an informa business

© 2021 Susan P. Gantt and Frances B. Carter

The right of Yvonne M. Agazarian, Susan P. Gantt and Frances B. Carter to be identified as authors of this work has been asserted by them in accordance with sections 77 and 78 of the Copyright, Designs and Patents Act 1988.

SCT® and Systems-Centered® are registered trademarks of the Systems-Centered Training and Research Institute, Inc., a non-profit organization.

SAVI® is a registered trademark of Claudia Byram & Frances Carter.

Unless indicated otherwise, all illustrations are copyrighted and owned by the Systems-Centered Training and Research Institute, Inc. (SCTRI) and are included here with permission of SCTRI.

Excerpt on page 189–191: Copyright © 2012. From *Small, large and median groups: The work of Patrick de Maré* by Lenn, R. & Stefano, K. Reproduced by permission of Taylor and Francis, a division of Informa plc.

Figures 8.2, 8.3 and 8.4 reproduced with permission of Jessica Kingsley Publishers Limited through PLSclear.

Figure 8.8 reproduced by kind permission of Phoenix Publishing House and originally appeared as Figure 3 in Gantt, S. P., & Agazarian, Y. M. (2007). Phases of system development in organizational work groups: The systems-centered approach for intervening in context. *Organisational & Social Dynamics* 7(2), 253–291.

British Library Cataloguing-in-Publication Data
A catalogue record for this book is available from the British Library

Library of Congress Cataloging-in-Publication Data
A catalog record for this book has been requested

ISBN: 978-0-367-64925-8 (hbk)
ISBN: 978-0-367-64924-1 (pbk)
ISBN: 978-1-003-12696-6 (ebk)

Typeset in Bembo
by Apex CoVantage, LLC

This book is dedicated to
anyone who is curious about living human systems,
all of us who care about how to work with differences differently,
the thousands of people who have learned together with us in our
SCT trainings and groups
and most especially our licensed SCT practitioners who have done
the work required to learn and practice SCT well enough to take
it into the world

Contents

Foreword

This book tells an engaging story about how models of complex phenomena are built, a story that nicely illuminates the reciprocal, iterative and ongoing process between careful observation and theory construction. It also reveals what those who undertake such an arduous task require in terms of courage in approaching what is not yet known, in remaining open to new experience, in a willingness to critique one's ideas and in persevering in efforts to understand and explain complicated relations among variables and constructs that form human living systems. Trying to fathom what happens in human groups, why it happens and what can be done to change what happens are tasks not for the faint of heart.

I've been a fan of Yvonne Agazarian and her lifelong team of colleagues ever since picking up her first book in 1981 precisely because of its intriguing title, *The Visible and Invisible Group*. This title, and, as it turned out, the novel ideas presented in this pioneering volume, spoke to my own intellectual struggles to make sense of group life and, more particularly, to bring together a depth view of the individual with a depth view of group psychology, an interest of mine that was borne of my graduate school experiences at Yale in the late 1960s. In that era, Yale Psychology and Psychiatry were at the forefront of studying and articulating the complex relations between the individual and the group, guided primarily by ego psychological (Edelson, 1970) and Kleinian object relations theoretical frameworks (Gibbard, Hartman, & Mann, 1974; Newton & Levinson, 1973). These classic writings, as well as the experiences generated from participating in the numerous Tavistock and Lewinian group relations conferences conducted at Yale in those days, have served as an important impetus in the awakening of my own curiosity about individual-in-the-group theory (Greene, 1982, 1983), a curiosity that has imbued my entire professional career and that has made reading this present volume so rewarding.

One can see the influences of these early theoretical efforts in the present volume: ideas about roles and role locks, about driving and restraining forces that, respectively, promote and inhibit goal attainment, about explicit and implicit goals and about the universal and ubiquitous dilemmas in group life in relating to authority and in developing peer relations. But this current work, the most recent in a long chain of theoretical and empirical contributions from the Agazarian team, has gone way beyond these foundational works, entering new territory by conceptualizing group life from a systems perspective. Their unique contributions, well summarized in Chapter 1 and elaborated in detail in the subsequent chapters, reveal the ever deepening and articulating of their thinking. I found their conceptual focus on the individual-becoming-a-group member, represented by their person-as-a-system model, particularly compelling precisely because it captures the ever-present dilemma of maintaining a sense of safety, familiarity and viability by attending exclusively to one's familiar self from the past versus the risking of this security to explore and discover, as Turquet (1975) so aptly put it, the skin of one's neighbor.

As substantive a contribution to building theoretical models as this volume is, this book is not just about theory. What helps to make theory robust are its links to empirical investigation and (in the case of psychological theories) to clinical practice. And this book well demonstrates vital connections to both of these enterprises. With regard to research, the singular accomplishment here is the construction of a classification system, dubbed SAVI, for analyzing communications in the group, not the content of the messages, but importantly what the messages serve in the way of furthering or obscuring information flow. Now I have no illusion that empirical research will answer all of the big questions about any complex phenomena of interest. One has only to look at the amassed empirical findings about the relationship of cohesion to outcome in group psychotherapy to understand the limitations of research. Despite decades of research on this relationship, most of what we can say is that generally a more cohesive group yields better outcomes. But the operative word in this rather tepid conclusion is "generally." We know little about the circumstances and conditions under which this relationship is maximized and when it can actually lead to negative results. And further, sadly, we still don't have a universal or shared definition of the cohesion construct.

Despite this not-so-optimistic view, empirical research such as the development and application of sophisticated process measures like SAVI does have heuristic value. Those studies (Agazarian & Simon, 1989; Simon & Agazarian, 2000) where its application serves to identify important patterns and relational dynamics can help both theorist and therapist in generating new hypotheses and new understandings of group life.

With regard to practice, I agree with the authors' assertion that the creation of the concept of functional subgrouping and its implementation in therapy and work groups is a vital procedure for helping these systems progress. In contrast to the natural regressive tendency in group life to form dysfunctional subgroups, either-or splits that serve to keep uncomfortable feelings and thoughts at arm's length, the conscious, intentional and proactive structuring of functional subgroups – where like-minded members can join together to explore (to apply one of the authors' engaging mantras) differences in the apparently similar and then also to discover similarities in the apparently different – potentiates the social organization towards greater differentiation and integration, hall-marks of progressive development.

Moreover, their ingenious techniques of linking and bridging by ask-ing members, first, to register their understanding of the previous member's remarks (and correcting misunderstandings if necessary via reality-checking) and then to conclude by asking whether "anybody else" joins with them so aptly counter the regressive tendencies in groups towards fragmentation or fusion.

Taken together, the career-long dedication of these authors to advancing our understanding of how groups work is truly impressive and inspiring. And their training of many others over the years – scholars, clinicians, researchers – holds promise that this systems view of group life will neither stagnate nor fade away but rather continue to develop and transform. In the spirit of SCT and functional subgrouping, I end by asking Agazarian, Gantt and Carter, did I get you right?

Les R. Greene, Ph.D.

References

Agazarian, Y. M., & Simon, A. (1989, February). The system for analyzing verbal interac-tion. In W. Piper (Chair), *Systems for viewing group interaction: Four perspectives on a therapy group in phase transition [open session]*. American Group Psychotherapy Association Annual Meeting, San Francisco, CA, US.

Edelson, M. (1970). *Sociotherapy and psychotherapy*. Chicago, IL: University of Chicago Press.

Gibbard, G. S., Hartman, J. J., & Mann, R. D. (1974). *Analysis of groups: Contributions to theory, research, and practice*. San Francisco, CA: Jossey-Bass.

Greene, L. R. (1982). Personal boundary management and social structure. In M. Pines & L. Rafaelson (Eds.), *The individual and the group: Boundaries and interrelations in theory and practice* (pp. 279–293). London, UK: Plenum Press.

Greene, L. R. (1983). On fusion and individuation processes in small groups. *International Journal of Group Psychotherapy*, *33*(1), 3–19. doi:10.1080/00207284.1983.11491741

Newton, P. M., & Levinson, D. J. (1973). The work group within the organization: A sociopsychological approach. *Psychiatry: Journal for the Study of Interpersonal Processes*, *36*(2), 115–142.

Simon, A., & Agazarian, Y. M. (2000). SAVI: The system for analyzing verbal interaction. In A. P. Beck & C. M. Lewis (Eds.), *The process of group psychotherapy: Systems for analyzing change* (pp. 357–380). Washington, DC: American Psychological Association.

Turquet, P. (1975). Threats to identity in the large group. In L. Kreeger (Ed.), *The large group: Dynamics and therapy* (pp. 87–144). London, UK: Constable.

Preface

It is fitting that we write this preface in the first days of 2020, as this book has taken almost the full decade to write. Yvonne Agazarian died in October 2017, a few months short of her 89th birthday. This book was dear to her and she worked hard on it. Yvonne had wanted to do an illustrated guide for the theory as long ago as 2000. Part of what took so long was Yvonne's embodiment of her theoretical commitment to test her ideas as well as continuing to take in new information and let the old framework fall apart until the new was integrated. Her other ongoing challenge was to find a way to take complex ideas and communicate them simply so others could understand too.

Both of us were involved with her work on the book in different ways, Fran in frequent discussions with Yvonne about theory and in her illustrations and Susan in theory and working with Yvonne as a writing partner. After Yvonne's death, we knew it was important for us to finish the book. We started off to finish "Yvonne's book," but in the process it became more than that; the book became ours too. We realized it really had to become ours for us to finish it. It has been a long journey and we have both developed in this process as we developed SCT and its theory in our writing and theorizing.

We could not have done this book without Kathy Lum, who contained the book, both of us and the whole of our team. Taylor Malone was an invaluable resource in her hands-on knowledge of Yvonne's previous work on the book and her archives, searching, organizing and knowing where and how to find the materials that Yvonne had compiled. Taylor and Miles Agag worked both separately and collectively, in editing, organizing and bringing our illustrations to life. Kathy, Taylor and Miles all knew and loved Yvonne, so they brought this full energy to the work they did to make this book happen.

Kaye Lott joined us later and contributed illustrations that captured the heart by taking our hand-drawn illustrations on small slips of paper and transforming them into computer images that contained the spirit of our drawings. We are also appreciative to Marianne Bentzen for her willingness to ensure that the neuroscience which we have integrated is accurate.

We also appreciated Kirk Larson's patience and support for both of us and for this book, including allowing the dining room to become our writing studio. We are also grateful for Claudia Byram's contributions as a member of our "thinking team" and quietly supporting our work all the way through. Thank you both.

Susan Gantt
Fran Carter
January 2020

Introduction

This book introduces systems-centered theory and its theory of living human systems in both words and illustrations. Most importantly, by defining the theory and its ideas and then illustrating these, this book builds a bridge for how to apply the ideas in the real world. Simply put, a theory is a way of thinking. This theory is a way of thinking about ourselves and others and the world around us. If a theory is to be useful, it will help us see something in a new way and, by seeing something from a new perspective, enable us to do something differently. We invite you to test out this theory by reading and thinking and feeling about the ideas and the illustrations and then checking to see whether anything different happens.

Systems-centered therapy and training (SCT) has widespread use in group psychotherapy, where it started (Gantt & Agazarian, 2017), as well as in the training of group therapists, consultation to organizations and teams, and in education. There are other SCT books listed in our appendix and a comprehensive list of SCT publications on our website (systemscentered.com) yet none that have the goal of illustrating SCT.

Equally important if not more so, this book describes how our leadership failure led to acting out scapegoating in our SCT large group. We took this to heart, as it was right at the heart of our theory. This led to a correction to our theory and practice and the development of our newer theory of the person-as-a-system. This book presents our newest theory and theorizing and discusses how we are now applying this new theory in practice.

The rest of this introduction to our illustrated guide is reprinted from a monograph that was published on the occasion of Yvonne's 80th birthday by the Systems-Centered Training and Research Institute (SCTRI), more than eight years before Yvonne died. This monograph, *Systems-Centered Theory and Practice: The Contribution of Yvonne Agazarian*, was "in honor and appreciation of the contributions Yvonne made with her theory of living human systems and its systems-centered practice, the founding of SCTRI, and in training and mentoring so many of us" (Gantt, 2010). The introduction to this manuscript is reprinted here with small edits, many of which Yvonne made herself, as she had selected this for the introduction to this book before she died in 2017.

[As Susan wrote in this introduction in 2010 when the monograph was published], I am enormously pleased in my role as director of SCTRI to be writing this brief overview of Yvonne's many contributions as theoretician, clinician, consultant and founder and director emeritus of SCTRI. I am also pleased personally to be writing this as Yvonne has impacted me and my work deeply. In this brief introduction, I hope to convey some of the highlights of Yvonne's contributions in developing a systems theory that can be applied with all living human systems, whether individual people, couples, families, organizational workgroups, organizations or even nations.

Taking to heart the task of applying systems thinking to group psychotherapy

As an earnest graduate student in the 1960s, Yvonne was appalled at the difficulty crossing between the language and constructs of individual psychoanalytic psychotherapy and those of group dynamics. Dave Jenkins, her professor at Temple University in Philadelphia, suggested to her she formulate a theory that would integrate both. This was the beginning impetus for what was much later to become a theory of living human systems. Another major catalyst began in 1980 when Yvonne joined the American Group Psychotherapy Association's (AGPA) General Systems Theory (GST) committee chaired by Helen Durkin. When this committee disbanded ten years later, Yvonne took to heart Jay Fiddler personally urging her to apply GST to the practice of group psychotherapy. Jay's charge stayed with Yvonne much as the project Dave Jenkins had proposed. By the early 1990s, Yvonne's theory of living human systems was rapidly taking shape and she articulated both the theory and practice in her 1997 book, *Systems-Centered Therapy for Groups* (Agazarian, 1997). This text still today remains the handbook for systems-centered training (SCT).

A theory of living human systems

Yvonne's theory of living human systems offers the most coherent and well-developed systems theory in its application to psychotherapy yet formulated. She describes it as a meta-theory in that a theory of living human systems can be used to understand and frame any method of change. Her theory of living human systems defines a "hierarchy of isomorphic systems that are energy-organizing, goal-directing and system-correcting" (Agazarian, 1997). Beginning with this one sentence statement of the theory, Yvonne then defined each of the constructs: hierarchy and isomorphy. Making definitions at each level of abstraction led to creating operational definitions from which hypotheses could be derived and from which the methods and techniques of systems-centered training were developed. As Yvonne says, each technique then tests the validity of the theory and the reliability of its practice. For example, hierarchy defines that a system always exists in the context of the system above it and is the context for the system below it in the hierarchy. In applying this idea, Yvonne recognized the enormous implications of always seeing a system or a subsystem in its context; that is, a system is never in isolation, it always exists in a context. Today SCT practitioners work actively with the understanding that whenever we take ourselves just personally, we have lost awareness of our context. Isomorphy is defined as similarity in structure and function for systems in a defined hierarchy. Structure is then operationally defined as boundaries that are permeable or impermeable to the flow of energy and information. Function is defined as the process by which living human systems survive, develop and transform through the process of discriminating and integrating differences, both differences in the apparently similar and similarities in the apparently different. The theory states that it is through the discrimination and integration of differences that systems survive, develop and transform from simpler to more complex. In the process of making this theory operational, the method of functional subgrouping was developed. Functional subgrouping is the hallmark of systems-centered practice and is possibly the contribution that has had the most impact on the field of group therapy and arguably may be the most influential and long-lasting of Yvonne's many contributions.

Functional subgrouping

Functional subgrouping is the heart of SCT practice. In fact, without functional subgrouping, a group is not an SCT group. Yvonne's introduction of the method of functional subgrouping as a conflict resolution method has gained wide acceptance from not only SCT practitioners but also from a broad theoretical array of practitioners, many of whom have integrated functional subgrouping into their practice. Many have recognized the enormous impact functional subgrouping has on weakening the acting out of scapegoating. Yvonne developed the method of functional subgrouping from her theory and her keen observations of groups that enabled her to discriminate functional from stereotyped or "basic assumptions" (Bion, 1961) subgrouping. To reiterate, the theory behind functional subgrouping is simple and profound: to the extent that a living human system discriminates and integrates its differences, it will survive, develop and transform. Functional subgrouping is a method that enables this process of discriminating differences in the apparently similar and similarities in the apparently different. In practice, any time there is a difference that is experienced as "too different," members choose which side of the conflict to explore in a subgroup with others who are also resonant with this side, and then in turn the second subgroup explores the other side of the conflict they are holding until there is an integration in the group-as-a-whole. Or, whenever someone says "yes, but," they are offered the option of exploring either the "yes" or the "but" with others that feel similarly. Yvonne's book, *A Systems-Centered Approach to Inpatient Group Psychotherapy* (Agazarian, 2001), provides an actual transcript of Yvonne working with a one-session group on an inpatient unit and illustrates functional subgrouping. Applying functional subgrouping to both therapy groups and training groups has enabled them to contain and explore group conflicts and the underlying group dynamics rather than acting out the dynamics by creating identified patients or scapegoats.

Driving and restraining forces in the phases of system development

Another major contribution is Yvonne's formulation of her phases of system development. Building on Bion (1961) and Bennis and Shepard's (1956) translation of Bion into a theory of group development, Yvonne applied the ideas of phases of development to systems and then integrated these phases of system development with Lewin's force field (1951). This enabled Yvonne to identify a predictable force field for each phase of system development, which then provided a map for change interventions. As Lewin would say, weakening the restraining forces releases the inherent drive to the goal. Weakening the restraining forces relevant to the system's phase of development then releases the driving forces towards development. For clinical practice, Yvonne then used this theoretical map to develop a hierarchy of defense modifications linked to the phases of system development, enabling therapists to tie their interventions to the context of the phase of the system's development. This hierarchy then guides a therapist in the process of change and more easily enables a modular approach to therapy when the reality constraints dictate short-term therapies.

The construct of role and moving from person to member

From early in her theorizing, Yvonne has worked with the construct of role as a bridge construct between the individual and the group. She introduced this idea in her first book, *The Visible and Invisible Group*, co-authored with her co-therapist Richard Peters (Agazarian & Peters, 1981). Later, using systems theory, Yvonne discriminated between the system of a person, which provides the energy for all living human systems, and the system of a member, which is the role that we take to relate to the goal of the context. Member role is the intervening subsystem between the person and the context. Most significantly, the first challenge is learning to take membership in one's self: learning to weaken the restraining forces or encapsulated internal roles that inhibit us from being more of ourselves. The next ongoing challenge is bringing our person system into our member role so that we can take up our roles in all the systems in which we are members with our heart and personal energy. Learning to take membership also weakens the human tendency to personalize that not only causes us anguish but also inhibits us from bringing our energy into the system and contributing to the group. As Yvonne says, learning to take things not just personally lowers the anguish for human beings. Similarly, learning to see the role, goal and context always lowers our human tendency to personalize.

Yvonne introduced the model of role, goal and context that is central in applying SCT to organizations. Learning to orient to the goal of the system context is critical in knowing how to take one's role to support the goal of one's context. This same model guides SCT practitioners in their work with couples, in which this model is introduced to the couple in terms of the four subsystems in a marriage, each of which has a goal and roles that implement the goal. For example, the parenting subsystem has the goal of raising children into functional adults or, as Yvonne often put it, "importing babies and exporting adults." The roles in this context are mother and father. Many marital conflicts are resolved when the couple understands that they are relating from incompatible system roles: like when one responds from the role of intimacy and the other from the role of bathing the baby (parenting) or balancing the checkbook (business system). Starting couples work with the clarity of these functional roles has enabled an important platform for the later work with the habitual roles that lock couples into redundant and dysfunctional patterns.

SAVI: the system for analyzing verbal interaction

In the 1960s, prior to developing SCT, Yvonne and her good friend and colleague Anita Simon developed a System for Analyzing Verbal Interaction (SAVI), a coding system for observing and coding verbal interactions (1967). The theory behind SAVI drew from Shannon and Weaver's (1964) theory of communication that postulated an inverse relationship between noise in the communication channel and the probability that the information in the channel would be received. SAVI also drew from Howard and Scott's theory of stress (1965), which viewed all behavior as moving towards or away from conflicts on the path to the goal, and Lewin's (1951) force field that translated the relationship between the verbal behaviors that approached the goal of the transfer of information and the restraining forces that avoided it. The SAVI system enables categorization of verbal communications into a frequency matrix that identifies communication patterns in a system and the likelihood of these patterns moving the system towards or away from successful communication, that is, the transfer of information. SAVI enabled a focus on "how" something is said, not "what" is said, identifying certain verbal behaviors (like ambiguous, redundant or contradictory talk) as restraining forces that make it difficult to hear "what" is said. SAVI and its theory not only provided a viable tool for training in effective communication and a research tool for learning to observe a system's communication patterns but also laid a foundation for the later development of SCT and its theory of living human systems. In a research project some years ago, Yvonne used SAVI to code communications in a therapy group and identified a flight pattern. Each time an individual would deviate from the flight norm, the group pattern would return to the norm. Most telling of the power of the system pattern was the moment in the group where there were three or four consecutive group communications that moved out of flight and the therapist's communication put the group back into flight. From this analysis, Yvonne became convinced that it is the group communication pattern that determines the problem-solving potential in the group, not the individuals, however skilled.

High on integrating

In all of her contributions, which are far greater than this brief summary allows, Yvonne's brilliance in integrating knowledge and other theories has enabled her to develop her highly integrative theory and systems-centered practice. To this day, on her 80th birthday, Yvonne continues in this work as she is actively integrating research from interpersonal neurobiology into systems-centered practice. This ongoing effort points to the heart of SCT. It is not a static theory or practice and is always developing and emerging. Though Yvonne's major focus is clinical and organizational development, many others whom she has trained have imported the work into education, professional coaching and managerial and leadership training.

Systems-Centered Training and Research Institute (SCTRI)

One other contribution is important to note. In 1995, Yvonne implemented her vision and founded SCTRI, a non-profit organization, using the theory and practice of SCT to build and develop the organization, that is, putting SCT into organizational practice. Developing this organization built on workshops held at Friends Hospital in Philadelphia as well as weekend workshops in Boston, Austin, Atlanta, San Francisco, London and York in the UK and ongoing New York and Philadelphia training groups. The nucleus of SCTRI was developed by a close group of four friends and colleagues, Claudia Byram, Fran Carter, Anita Simon and Yvonne, who met regularly, exploring how to make the theory practical and to design training experiences for an ever-widening interest. The four, later called the Policy Action Group or PAG, met weekly, and after one workshop in the early 1990s the idea of becoming an organization surfaced in the debriefing period. There were immediately two subgroups, one excited about "organizing" and the other determined to organize without any hierarchy! Yvonne and PAG were determined not to replicate traditional organizations and instead followed the idea of "laying the paths" by following where the members trod using the theory and methods as a guide. This experiment has led to an active international organization of 230 members, many of whom are in SCT training in one of the nine training groups in the US or one of the four in Europe and who subgroup by telephone to do the work of the organization. Many of these members and others also gather once a year for the SCT annual conference, which just celebrated its tenth anniversary.[1] SCTRI was recently selected for the 2010 Award for Outstanding Contributions in Education and Training in the Field of Group Psychotherapy given by the National Registry of Certified Group Psychotherapists of AGPA.

Courage to bring in differences

Along the way of developing her theory, Yvonne has provided an important model by having the courage to say what she knows and to speak the unspeakable. Two episodes illustrate this well. In 1989, Yvonne was an invited discussant for Sampson and Weiss, who were invited lecturers for the Slavson Memorial Lecture at AGPA (Agazarian & Gantt, 2000). In preparing her remarks, Yvonne linked her systems theory to Sampson and Weiss' idea of the pathogenic belief, towards the goal of generalizing their work to group dynamics. In doing this, Yvonne recognized the pathogenic belief inherent in psychoanalysis and individual therapy, that the first pathogenic belief is that the patient is the center of the world, which masks a deeper pathogenic belief that the analyst is. As she had trained as a psychoanalyst, this recognition seemed heresy to Yvonne as she recognized that therapy can actually encourage self-centeredness at the expense of seeing the larger system context. Yet she held fast to what she had seen as she described in her remarks how group therapy can weaken the pain that comes from an "egocentric focus."

Or similarly, when on a panel with Yalom in 1992 at AGPA where excerpts of his tapes were shown and discussed, Yvonne used "who to whom," which tracks who is speaking to whom and SAVI to code the communication patterns in the group excerpts (Agazarian, 1992; Agazarian & Gantt, 2000). In both excerpts, the pattern was "communication to a deviant." In the first, the group elected an identified patient for the therapist to cure and, in the second, a scapegoat for the group to blame. Yvonne then described how a systems-centered approach would differ, by encouraging functional subgrouping to explore the roles that were being enacted. Both of these experiences are described in more detail in Yvonne's 2000 book, *Autobiography of a Theory*, co-authored with Susan Gantt. In this book, Yvonne traces the steps along the way to developing her theory and the moments and influences in her life that contributed to her work.

Yvonne's favorite of her books, *Systems-Centered Practice: Selected Papers on Group Psychotherapy* (2006), brings together published articles from 1987–2002 that illustrate Yvonne's theory and the stepping stones in her thinking as she is developing it. In fact, her own summary of this book describes the theoretical challenge to which she has devoted her work: "The book covers various stages in my attempts to solve the problem represented by the fact that, though group dynamics are different from the dynamics of individuals, yet group is often defined as the sum of individual dynamics" (Agazarian, 2006, p. 1).

Recognition

As Yvonne's theory strongly emphasizes, the challenge of introducing a difference is not easy as human beings tend to close their boundaries to differences that are too different. SCT does introduce radical differences. It is a tribute to the clarity of Yvonne's theorizing and apprehensive understandings that, in spite of the radical differences she has introduced, she has gained wide recognition. For example, she was invited to deliver the 12th Annual Foulkes Memorial Lecture in 1989, was recognized as a fellow in the American Psychological Association, and was named a distinguished fellow in AGPA.[2] She also served for ten years on the board of the International Association of Group Psychotherapy and for eight years as the first director of SCTRI. There have been many highlights in Yvonne's prolific contributions and many significant moments, but none more telling than her recognition as Group Psychologist of the Year in 1997 by Division 49 of the American Psychological Association:

> For her involvement in research, publication, teaching and training. She exemplifies the finest in scholarship in the discipline of psychology. As a group psychologist, she has contributed to expanding our knowledge of the boundaries between clinical and social psychology with the investigation of living human systems and systems-centered group and individual therapy. Her considerable body of work illustrates the highest blend of creativity and learning.

Yvonne's influence is far-reaching. As a group theorist and practitioner, few have offered the coherent theory and practice that she has developed and introduced, the training program that she pioneered, the training and research institute that she founded, and the books and articles she has authored. Yet as important to Yvonne are the thousands whom she has trained directly as well as the thousands whom other licensed systems-centered practitioners have trained and the even larger number who have read her many books and articles worldwide.[3] It is also valuable to note the strong personal connections she forms with those she teaches and trains: some may think this paradoxical as Yvonne has so strongly emphasized the system and the importance of learning to shift from person to member and take membership in one's person. Yet it is the resources of us as people that are the energy and life force in living human systems and, as those who know Yvonne well know, the person energy is the life force for any living human system.

For myself, from my first experience with Yvonne in the early 1990s at an AGPA meeting in San Antonio, where I learned to work with the group rather than struggle internally with myself, I recognized that Yvonne offered a theory and method that are unique and revolutionary. Yvonne has been the most significant mentor I have had and my personal and professional association with her ranks as the most influential of my life and, *most importantly*, there are many others who would say this as well. For Yvonne lives as she teaches and builds the relational system with whomever she is relating. This may be her greater legacy to us all, to take up the call of membership and citizenship wherever we are, albeit with ourselves, our loved ones, our colleagues, our organizations, our countries and our world.

This book is Yvonne's last one, and she spent the last years of her life working on it. In its finished form, the book is written by the three of us and would not be possible without all of us, as we all have made vital contributions to it and the newer theory of the person system that is introduced here.

We start in Chapter 1 by introducing the operational definitions of a theory of living human systems (TLHS) and some of the systems-centered methods that bring the ideas into practice. This chapter also holds the heart of this book's original goal, using illustrations to help bring SCT theory to life and to playfully discover how to go from words to illustrations and then back again as we put these ideas into practice in the real world!

Chapter 2 focuses on energy in living human systems and discusses how a TLHS has operationally defined energy as equivalent to information. Energy/information fuels all living human systems. We describe with illustrations how a system's energy is organized, directed towards its goals and corrected. We also introduce the force field to diagnose the likelihood of the system reaching its primary goals of survival, development and transformation as well as its secondary goals in mastering its problem or task in the environment.

Chapter 3 tells the story of the transformation in our theory precipitated by our conference large group in 2013 where we inadvertently regressed to acting out scapegoating. As SCT is all about integrating differences rather than avoiding them or scapegoating them, this was an eye-opener for us and an important turning point that enabled us to make a correction in our theory. This chapter describes the large group enactment, the subsequent theoretical correction, and presents our new theory picture, a person-as-a-system illustration that emerged from our correction.

Chapter 4 elaborates the theory that our new person-as-a-system illustration enabled us to develop, in seeing roles as role-systems. We describe how we deepened our understanding of our new illustration by elaborating it using the constructs of our theory. The implications that then emerged resulted in further refinements and conceptualization of how energy is vectored between and within role-systems.

Chapter 5 describes our discovery of how to use our new illustration as a map to help us identify our role-system by its role-system output, both how we talk and how we walk or stand or sit or nonverbally communicate our role-system of origin. Using this "map" has also enabled us to explore the territory of ourselves and our groups in new ways and to deepen our understanding of roles and role locks by viewing them from this map. We also introduce here what we discovered that had been implicit, and that is that our person-as-a-system map can also be understood more generically as a role-systems map that can be applied in any context.

In Chapter 6, we explore the implications our role-systems map has had on our understanding of our inner-person systems, both the affiliative/attachment roles and our social roles. Importantly, we present how our role-systems map has helped us deepen our understanding of working with inner-person survivor role-systems.

In Chapter 7, we discuss applications of using our role-systems map in our clinical, organizational and training contexts. This map has helped us assess readiness for change and has impacted our training of therapists and consultants in recognizing how the goals of different systems relate to different contexts, for example, the therapy system goal is developing the inner-person while training and organizational consultation focuses on inter-person goals. We also introduce our new phylogenetic role protocol. We end with a return to SAVI and our early theorizing (1960s) with Anita Simon to explore integrating our role-system theory with the SAVI Grid.

In Chapter 8, we highlight some of the important theoretical influences on SCT's work with phases as well as the work of colleagues that has enriched our theorizing around phases. We also recount how we used SAVI to identify system phases and how it has been the underpinning for our theoretical conceptualization of SCT phases and our work in operationally defining them as a force field. We then focus on how we are now using theory to integrate the phases of development chart and its force field map as a guide to our practice. We end with discussing how we have linked our phase model with our role-systems map.

In Chapter 9, we build on the theoretical work described in Chapter 8 and introduce SCT's phases of system development in more detail. We also elaborate and illustrate how we have used the force field to operationally define each phase of system development. Lastly, we integrate our new role-systems map with our model of the phases of system development.

Notes

1 Our next SCT conference in 2021 will be our 21st annual conference.
2 Yvonne was also awarded a Presidential Citation from the American Psychological Association in 2014 "for her pioneering work in developing a theory of living human systems and its systems-centered practice, and for training thousands of practitioners worldwide."
3 As of the time of this writing, more than 100 books, chapters and articles have been published by Yvonne and other SCT practitioners and students of SCT.

References

Agazarian, Y. M. (1992, February). *The use of two observation systems to analyze the communication patterns in two videotapes of the interpersonal approach to group psychotherapy*. [Based on I. D. Yalom "Understanding group psychotherapy" (videotape). Pacific Grove, CA: Brooks-Cole]. Panel on "Contrasting views of representative group events", American Group Psychotherapy Association Annual Meeting, New Orleans, LA, US.

Agazarian, Y. M. (1997). *Systems-centered therapy for groups*. New York, NY: Guilford Press. Reprinted in paperback (2004). London, UK: Karnac Books.

Agazarian, Y. M. (2001). *A systems-centered approach to inpatient group psychotherapy*. London, UK and Philadelphia, PA: Jessica Kingsley.

Agazarian, Y. M. (2006). *Systems-centered practice: Selected papers on group psychotherapy*. London, UK: Karnac Books.

Agazarian, Y. M., & Gantt, S. P. (2000). *Autobiography of a theory: Developing a theory of living human systems and its systems-centered practice*. London, UK: Jessica Kingsley.

Agazarian, Y. M., & Peters, R. (1981). *The visible and invisible group*. London, UK: Routledge & Kegan Paul. Reprinted in paperback (1987). London, UK: Karnac Books.

Bennis, W. G., & Shepard, H. A. (1956). A theory of group development. *Human Relations*, *9*(4), 415–437. doi:10.1177/001872675600900403

Bion, W. R. (1961). *Experiences in groups*. London, UK: Tavistock.

Gantt, S. P. (2010). Introduction: The achievements and influence of Yvonne Agazarian. In Y. M. Agazarian & SCTRI (Eds.), *Systems-centered theory and practice: The contribution of Yvonne Agazarian* (pp. vii–xviii). Livermore, CA: WingSpan Press. Reprint (2011). London, UK: Karnac Books.

Gantt, S. P., & Agazarian, Y. M. (2017). Systems-centered group therapy. *International Journal of Group Psychotherapy*, *67*(sup1), S60–S70. doi:10.1080/00207284.2016.1218768

Howard, A., & Scott, R. A. (1965). A proposed framework for the analysis of stress in the human organism. *Journal of Applied Behavioral Science*, *10*, 141–160. doi:10.1002/bs.3830100204

Lewin, K. (1951). *Field theory in social science*. New York, NY: Harper & Row.

Shannon, C. E., & Weaver, W. (1964). *The mathematical theory of communication*. Urbana, IL: University of Illinois Press.

Simon, A., & Agazarian, Y. M. (1967). *SAVI: Sequential analysis of verbal interaction*. Philadelphia, PA: Research for Better Schools.

Chapter 1

Illustrating the nuts and bolts of a theory of living human systems

A theory of living human systems (TLHS) defines a hierarchy of isomorphic systems that are energy-organizing, goal-directing and self-correcting. Don't get put off by this sentence or go away. At first, hearing this definition can be a bit daunting, yet the rest of this entire book is about making the meaning of this sentence clearer. By bringing these words to life through illustrations, we can experiment with what it is like to see ourselves and others through the lens of this theory.

This book is a guide to a TLHS. It defines each of the words in this statement and illustrates these ideas. The illustrations help us both apprehend the theory *and* build a link from theory to systems-centered practice. Importantly, these illustrations have helped us not only formulate the theory but also translate the theory into practice and make it possible to see things and do things in the real world differently from the way we saw or did them before. Yvonne's theorizing (and consequently that of all systems-centered therapy and training [SCT] practitioners) was heavily influenced by Lewin (1951a), who said, "there is nothing so practical as a good theory" (p. 169).

For Yvonne, as a deductive reasoner as many theoreticians are, it has always been necessary to find a sign or a symbol or a picture that can build the bridge between the intuitive sense that she knew something important and the words that will describe what it is so that she could communicate to others. Once having found a symbol that seems to represent the idea, she could then keep it in her mind (or in front of her on paper) and think about and explore what it represents.

For many of us, a picture is indeed worth a thousand words. Our boundaries are often more open to visual information than words, and the visual can help us access a different part of ourselves. Putting an idea, an intuition, or apprehensive information into words is a vital journey we must take, to make use of both the nonverbal and verbal information we all have available to us as resources in living our lives and in working with others to live and work with less of the anguish of personalizing. Going forward in this book, we put pictures into words and words into pictures. By illustrating a theory of living human systems, we hope to make it easier to understand the ideas and help shift from thinking about people to thinking about systems and back again, from thinking about systems to thinking about people. What is new is taking to heart the work of illustrating our theory as a bridge to more theorizing and also as a pathway to practice and everyday life.

Why thinking systems matters

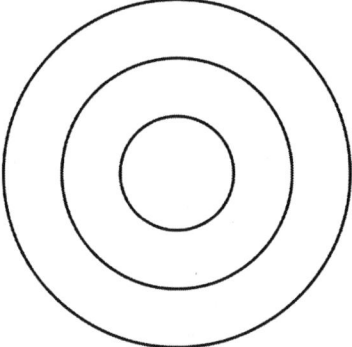

Figure 1.1

This chapter focuses on "thinking systems" as a different way of thinking about people. A TLHS gives us a common language to think about a person as well as the environments or contexts within which we all live. System dynamics powerfully influence us as people or, as we say often in SCT, who and how we are at any moment has as much, and likely more, to do with our system context than our own dynamics. Seeing the system dynamics of individuals, subgroups and the whole group helps give us an understanding of not only our own experiences but also our experience as part of our larger environment or context.

A new language and a new way of thinking

Why is it worth learning a new language and a new way of thinking about group psychotherapy? Systems ideas are not new; they have long been popular. There are many scholars in the field who have addressed system ideas and a whole committee in the American Group Psychotherapy Association (AGPA) that devoted many years attempting to find ways of applying systems thinking to group psychotherapy. Applying systems thinking to our own disciplines is not an easy exercise, but we propose it as a useful one. It has provided us with perspectives that allow us to enrich our vision about and our practice in groups, individual therapy and couples therapy and in consultation to professionals who are involved as change agents in many organizational, educational and social settings.

Building a theory means finding the words that will express the idea: a TLHS defines a hierarchy of isomorphic systems. We then take the important step to define each word in this statement. As soon as we have defined each word, we can make an operational definition. An operational definition is like a blueprint for putting the idea contained in the word into practice. Operational definitions lead to hypotheses, and hypotheses lead to testing in the real world. This process is how systems-centered therapy and systems-centered training were developed from a TLHS.

Yet these words are only part of the story. It has always been for us that using images and illustrations helps us elaborate our apprehensive sense and allows us, in turn, to apprehend from our illustrations. We start first with the image of a circle. This image has been essential to the heart of how SCT sees the system and how it organizes the flow of energy in and out. The circle was our first step to give us an illustration that expresses the idea of a system itself.

The system as a circle

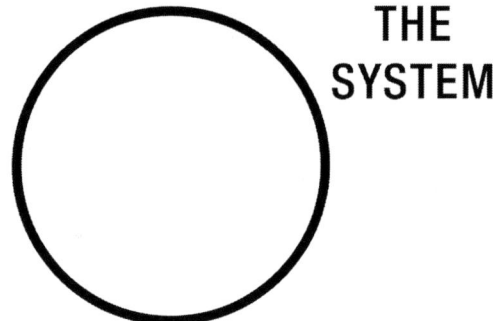

Figure 1.2

We have used the drawing of a circle to make the bridge between the word "system," which is an abstract idea, and visualizing the properties of a system that are important to understand if the idea of a system is to be of use to us. A person, a couple, a family, a team, an organization and a country are all living human systems and can all be represented by a circle.

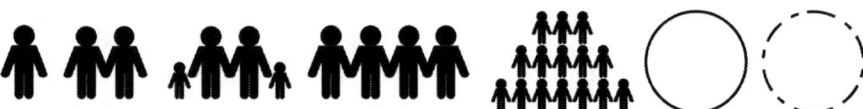

Figure 1.3

When we look at the family silhouettes in Figure 1.3, we start to think about mom and dad and even gender roles. When we shift to think of the family system as a *circle*, we can then start to think about all the things that can happen when we see a system, any system, as a circle, and as an abstraction. For example, if the circle represented a therapy group, we can think about how to best draw the circle of the group. We could draw a closed circle for a closed group or a circle with dotted lines for a drop-in group. Thinking about the circle and how open or closed it is helps us think about the group boundary and it might also give us ways to think about how each group functions. So simply by drawing a circle to represent a group, we have started to think about how group boundaries impact function. This gives a good sense of how illustrations have helped us develop our theorizing. Before we elaborate on boundaries, we shift to introducing the nuts and bolts of our theory.

The nuts and bolts of a TLHS

We start with an overview of a TLHS and follow with the methods for SCT that have been derived from the operational definitions of its theoretical constructs. A TLHS includes definitions, some of which you will recognize from general systems theory (von Bertalanffy, 1968) and others of which we defined in the process of developing a TLHS (Agazarian, 1997).

Yvonne was often fond of saying (with a smile on her face) that the overall sentence which defines a TLHS represented her life's work and only took about 30–40 years to develop. Returning to this same sentence that we used at the beginning of this chapter, the two main constructs of the theory are identified here in bold type. These constructs and the variables (in italics) are the fundamental building blocks of a TLHS upon which SCT has been developed.

> A theory of living human systems defines a **hierarchy** of **isomorphic** systems that are *energy-organizing*, *goal-directing* and *self-correcting*.

Defining the constructs and variables in systems language has given us a common language to explore the relationship between individual systems and group systems. Without a common language (which a systems approach provides), we would have no alternative but to use psychodynamic language to describe individuals and group dynamic language to define groups. This would be a significant liability as without a common language, there are no common variables with which to link the two for research.

Hierarchy

We start with the construct of *hierarchy*. Hierarchy defines that a system exists in the context of a larger system and is the context for a smaller system. With

Hierarchy

Systems come in threes. Every system exists in the context of the system above and is the context for the system below.

The circle exists in the context of other circles.

Context

System-centered contexts define a recursive triad of isomorphic systems in a defined hierarchy.

Every system always exists in the context of the larger system above it and is itself the context for the smaller system below it.

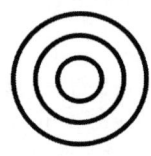
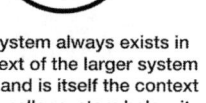
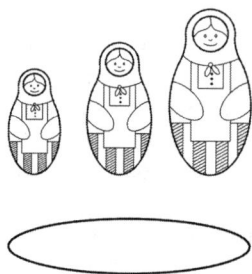

Figure 1.4

this definition, all living human systems always exists in a context and never in isolation.

In SCT, hierarchy means always thinking of a system as a triad of systems. Seeing systems as triads easily translates systems thinking to individuals, sub-groups and groups. Thinking systems requires thinking context. Like a set of nested dolls, each system exists not only as the system itself, but in the context of the system above and as the context for the system below. We have defined the basic SCT hierarchy or triad as the person, member and system-as-a-whole.

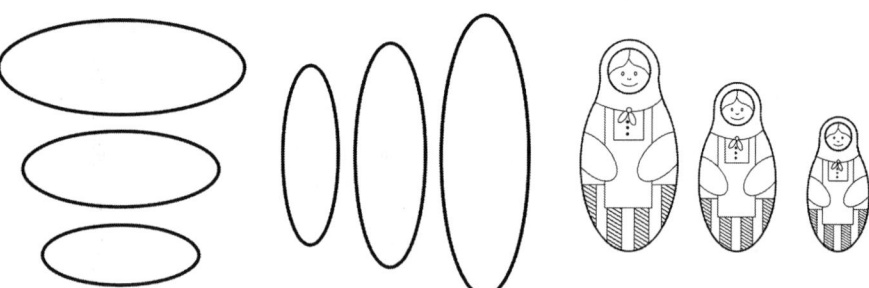

Figure 1.5

Without thinking hierarchy, we tend to see a system as just itself, stand-ing alone instead of belonging to a nested system hierarchy which keeps us thinking context. This perspective also has an important implication for thinking about how to influence change through the middle circle in a triad of systems as the middle circle shares its boundaries with the smaller circle and the larger circle.

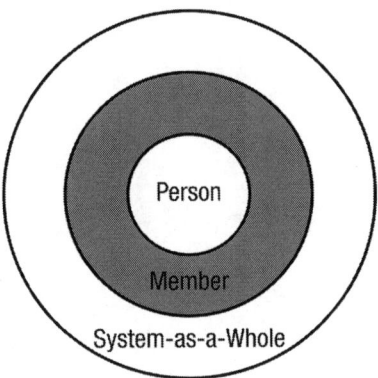

Figure 1.6

Thinking theory, we would hypothesize that interventions to the subgroup or member system as the middle system will probably have the greatest impact simultaneously on both the person and the larger group system or system-as-a-whole, as they both share contiguous boundaries with the middle member system.

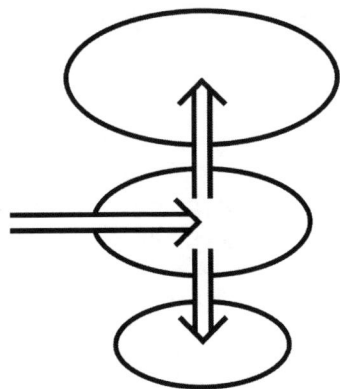

Figure 1.7

Isomorphy

From a hierarchy of nested systems, we then say that whatever one learns about any one system in the nested systems will apply to every system in the hierarchy of systems. This defines *isomorphy*, which means that all systems in the hierarchy are similar and equivalent in structure and function. Practically, this means that if you discover how to increase the efficiency of one living human system (like discovering methods to increase communication across a boundary), these same methods can be used to increase the efficiency in communication across all the boundaries of the systems in a defined hierarchy.

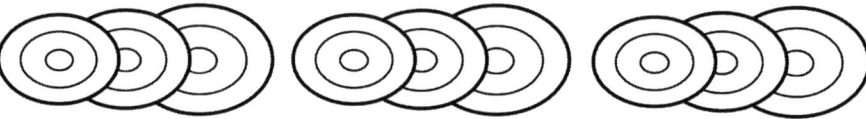

Person - Member - Group   Member - Group - Clinic   Group - Clinic - Hospital

Figure 1.8

We start with a simple chart of isomorphy, which means similarity in system structure and function for systems in a defined hierarchy.

Isomorphy Systems are similar in structure and function and different in different contexts.	
Structure Systems-centered structure defines boundaries in space, time and context that are potentially permeable to energy and information.	**Function** Systems-centered function is to survive, develop and transform by discriminating and integrating differences and similarities.

Structure and function

Next in our theorizing, we need to define structure and function. This means applying systems language to create theoretical definitions for how systems are structured to organize energy and how they function to self-correct. Structure links to the variable of energy-organizing, function links to the variable of self-correcting, and both variables link to our overall theory statement.

Defining structure as boundaries

Going back to our illustration of the circle is useful here. The line of the circle is a structure that defines its boundary.

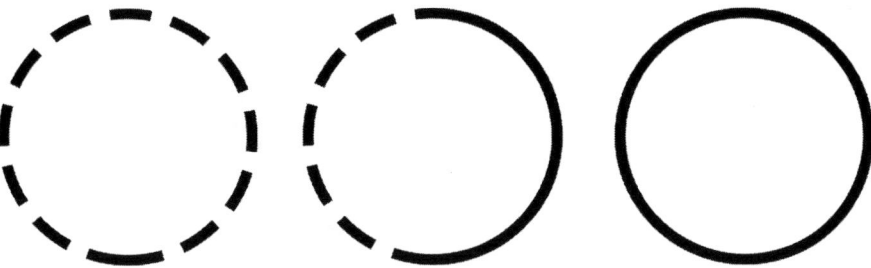

Figure 1.9

Looking again at our circles: if we look at this illustration (see Figure 1.9), we can see that the circle can be represented by a dashed line, a solid line or both or almost not there at all. This illustrates how a system can have open boundaries (dashes), closed boundaries (solid) or both and is potentially permeable. In other words, system boundaries can open and close. It is the representation of the boundary permeability that lets us know whether a system is open or closed.

The line is also a boundary that defines what is inside the circle or system and what is outside it.

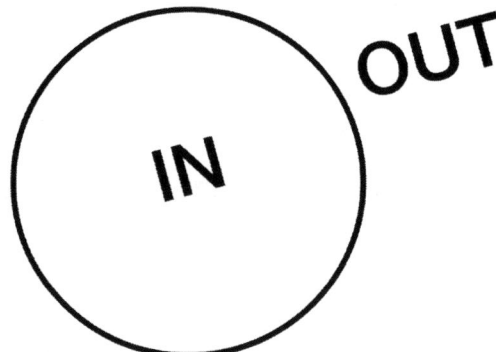

Figure 1.10

Open systems survive, develop and transform through an integration of the information that crosses the boundary. Closed systems survive at the expense of development and transformation as no new information can enter the system. Systems can be too open (flooded with more energy/information faster than the system can integrate), too closed (no energy/information can cross the boundary) or appropriately permeable (able to open and close dependent on the system's readiness to take in new information or differences).

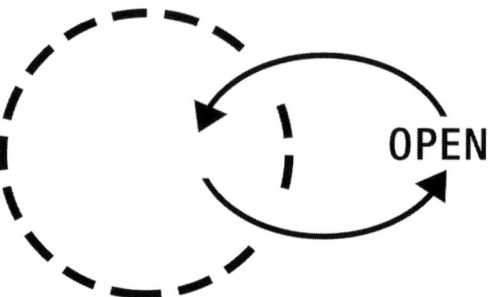

Figure 1.11

Appropriately permeable boundaries make for open systems. In this illustration, the boundary is permeable, and the arrows represent the flow of energy, or information in communications that can cross the boundaries between systems. The boundaries let the outside in and the inside out. The advantage of open systems is that they can receive communications from the outside and send communications out from the inside. Thus, the system is open to communication exchanges between itself and its environmental context. However, if too much information enters the system at one time or the flow of information is too fast, the system will not be able to integrate the information and reorganize and instead will become disorganized or close.

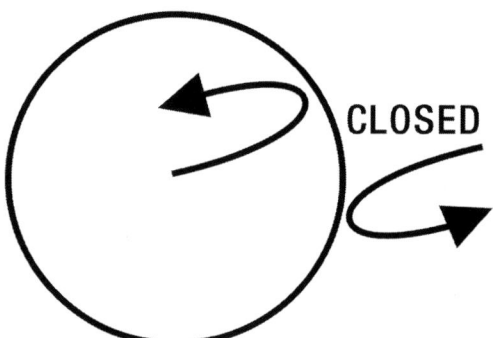

Figure 1.12

Closed boundaries make closed systems. In this illustration, the system is closed. The boundary keeps the inside in and the outside out. The advantage of a closed system is that it allows new information that has entered the system to be organized. It is useful to be able to "stop and think." Another advantage is that it protects the current organization within the system. The disadvantage to a closed system is that it cannot take in new information necessary for development. Think about the difference between when our mind is open versus when we have a closed mind.

It is important for system boundaries to be appropriately permeable to information both within the system itself and between the system and the larger system context or environment. In the communication with the outside context, new information is necessary for development, orientation to reality and problem-solving.

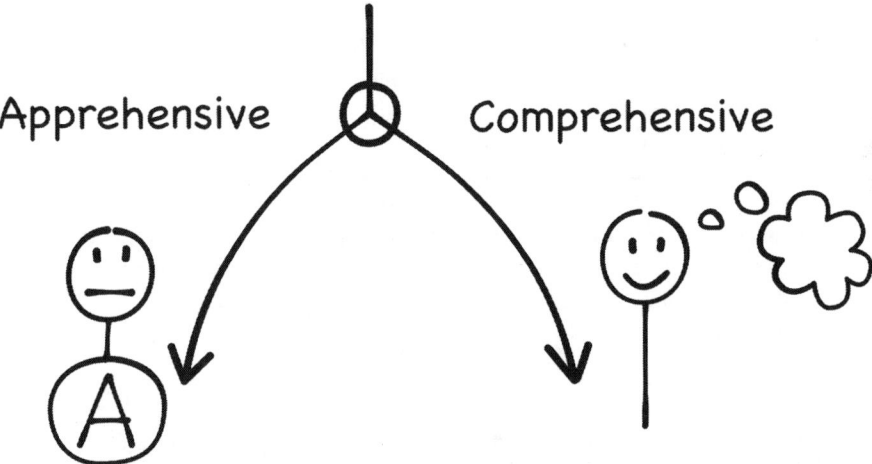

Apprehensive **Comprehensive**

Figure 1.13

In oneself, when our internal boundaries are open to both our comprehensive (cognitive thinking) and apprehensive (intuitive emotional) information, we can work with our common sense. When our boundary is closed, we either live overdetermined by our thoughts without the feeling that will give us a sense of meaning or we live in the back-and-forth of our emotional life without a practical link to reality-testing and problem-solving.

To recap, SCT defines structure as system boundaries that organize system energy and open and close to titrate energy.

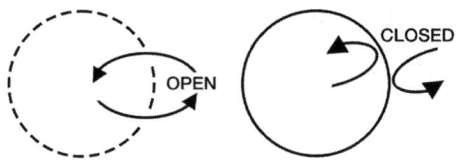

Figure 1.14

Defining function as discriminating and integrating differences

We started by defining function as the process of discriminating and integrating differences in the energy/information in the system. This is important in that the challenge for all living human systems is that differences introduce conflict. From our systems view, all living human systems need differences to develop and transform over time. Yet differences are not easy for us. As a human species, we do not like differences. Differences (when they are different enough) are destabilizing to what we already know. When there is a difference, the system has to disorganize in order to reorganize with the integration of the new information in the difference.

SCT has defined that living human systems *function* to survive, develop and transform from simpler to more complex through the process of discriminating and integrating differences, differences in the apparently similar and similarities in the apparently different. This is very useful as we can then think about the potential for survival, development and transformation by looking at what a system is doing with differences. In Figure 1.15, the first picture shows the "difference" being isolated, and the second picture shows all the communication towards the difference. This "communication pattern to a deviant" could be scapegoating the difference or care-taking it. The third picture shows the difference being joined by those who are similar and the last, how the difference is integrated in the whole system.

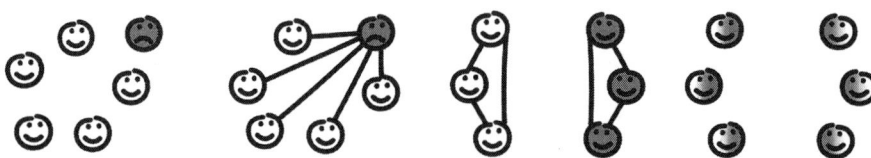

Figure 1.15

Discriminating differences in the apparently similar is the first and often the easiest step to take. Seeing differences in what seemed "just similar" develops an ability to separate and differentiate. For example, when we ask ourselves, "how is the present different from the past?", we can separate from the past and orient to our present.

When systems discriminate similarities in the apparently different, the system develops an ability to integrate new experience and individuate. When we do this, we discover that "they" are not so different from us; someone else actually feels the same way we do!

Putting function into practice

In developing the theory, we kept revisiting the illustration of seeing a system as a hierarchy of three separate but interconnected systems (see Figure 1.5) We continued to note that the member system is the only system that shares its boundaries with both the person system and the system-as-a-whole. We kept recognizing the unique position that the member system occupied in the triad of systems. Finally, our insight came! The implication of understanding the potential influence of the member system on the system-as-a-whole as well as the person due to its location in the triad revolutionized how we thought about how to direct our interventions. Before adopting a systems orientation, we had vectored our interventions to the person. However, from a systems perspective, interventions to the member system can influence all three systems at once. Thus, therapeutic interventions to the member system would be potentially more powerful than interventions to either the central person system or the system-as-a-whole.

This insight was great in theory! However, at the beginning we did not have the slightest idea how to implement it in practice. We already knew from our work with groups that group dynamics were a powerful influence on the individual dynamics, and we were already successful in reducing the tendency to scapegoat or create identified patients to contain the splits inherent in group dynamics. Yet we did not have a method which would enable the integration of differences at the system level.

In fact, it was many years before we perceived what had been there all along: the phenomenon of transitory subsystems that develop in the member system as members came together spontaneously around similarities and separated again around differences. These "subgroups" were already recognized in the field and were often given a bad name when they contributed to flight and fight dynamics. What we recognized when we began to study subgrouping was how subgroups could be both a driving and a restraining force. Seeing this helped us see how we could develop methods that would change them from dysfunctional to functional subgroups! This is now taken for granted in SCT as our core method of functional subgrouping. In SCT, people develop as they become members of subgroups. Subgroups are transient subsystems. These systems can be systems of dyads or small groups or large or larger groups. They can also be subgroups inside the system of the self, like exploring two sides of a question or exploring two sides (or subgroups) inside us when we have a conflict or a question or exploring both sides of what SCT calls a fork-in-the-road. Functional subgroups *function* to discriminate and integrate differences. Stereotyped or nonfunctional subgroups ignore, stereotype or attack differences.

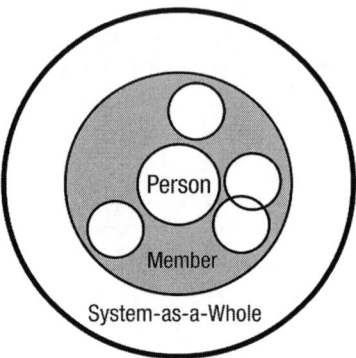

Figure 1.16

More on transitory subgroups

In SCT, we now define two types of subgroups: stereotyped subgroups and functional subgroups. Stereotyped subgroups come together around similarities and separate around differences. Stereotyped subgroups often scapegoat differences, which explains the tendency in systems to create the identified patient or scapegoat in a group or inside ourselves to attack our own thoughts or feelings or reactions.

In contrast, SCT encourages members to form functional subgroup systems, within themselves and with others, with the goal of recognizing differences and integrating them rather than scapegoating them. We will revisit this in Chapter 3, on the topic of "our wake-up call," where we describe how we inadvertently created both identified patients and scapegoats in our 2013 conference large group!

The functional subgrouping system

Unique to systems–centered practice is our norm of developing functional subgrouping right from the beginning of every SCT group. Functional subgrouping is a method that enables the discrimination and integration of differences in contrast to the natural human tendency to form the stereotyped subgroups that split away from differences and create identified patients or scapegoats to contain and isolate the differences.

Subgroup subsystems

Subgroups are those transitory subsystems that come into existence when members join around a common theme and disappear again when members no longer have something in common. Discovering how subgroups could become a driving force is perhaps SCT's most important contribution to working with groups. The one fundamental principle in a TLHS and SCT is that any system will survive, develop and transform through the ongoing process of discriminating and integrating differences. We see this as potentially revolutionary. For example, recognizing and accepting differences would solve the human tendency to ignore, attack, isolate or "take care of" those who hold a difference, instead of seeing what we have in common with them so that we can join them and discover how we can use the differences as a resource. From early in my work, I (Yvonne) had been looking for a solution to the tendency that all groups seemed to have of creating the identified patient in the flight phase and the scapegoat in the fight phase. Then I suddenly saw something unseen and obvious: scapegoating in groups is a subgrouping phenomenon!

The clear circle (see Figure 1.17) is being ostracized by the shaded circles.

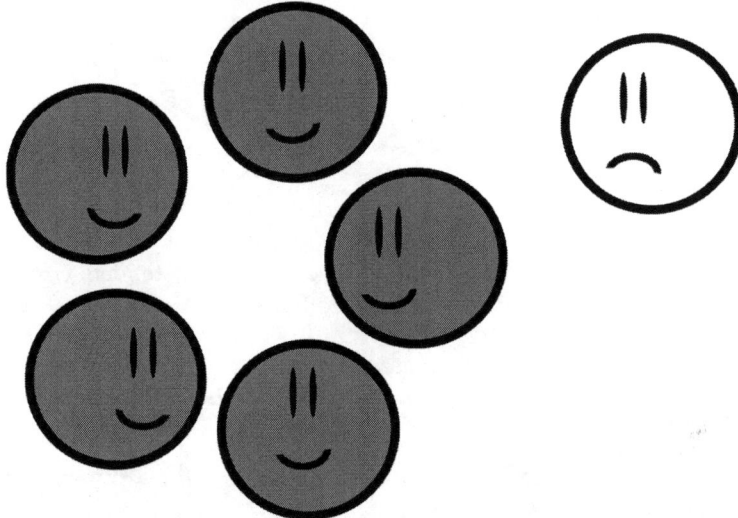

Figure 1.17

In the next set of circles (see Figure 1.18), those who are "similar" (coded as S in the figure) cluster together. In the second picture in this figure, the similar (S) focus on the difference (D), typical of a communication to deviant pattern like creating an identified patient or a scapegoat. In the third picture, the similars only talk and relate to each other and ignore the difference, and in the last of the pictures in this figure, the difference has been extruded.

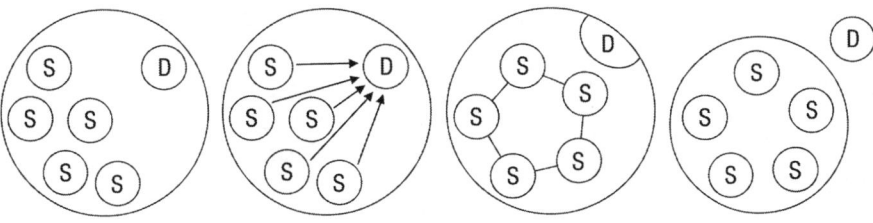

Figure 1.18

Putting functional subgrouping into practice

The question then became, how could we as leaders influence subgroups so that they could be used to put the theory into practice? The answer turned out to be what we now call functional subgrouping. Subgrouping functionally reverses the tendency to split around differences and fight over them and substitutes methods that require members to join around their similarities and explore them.

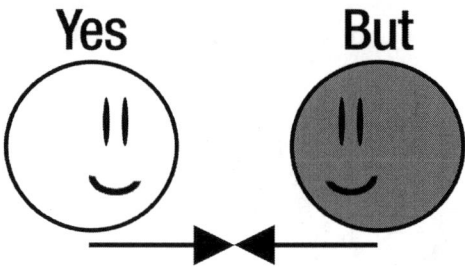

Figure 1.19

The solution turned out to be as simple as changing the tendency to split by saying "yes, but" to building on what each other says instead with a "yes, and."

Figure 1.20

Functional subgrouping is functional! When a subgroup joins around similarities, the members more easily accept and integrate just noticeable differences within the subgroup of similarities. As these small differences are integrated, the system itself develops more complexity. As different subgroups integrate various group differences, there comes a point in time when the similarities between the subgroups become more interesting than the differences. When that happens, integration has taken place between subgroups and within the

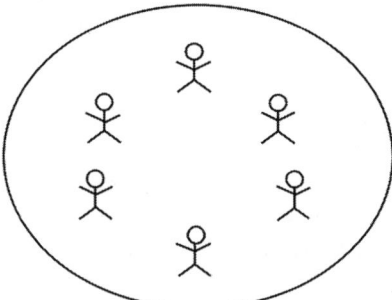

Time 1: Group comes together

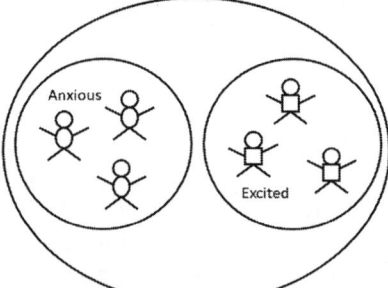

Time 2: A difference emerges – represented here by round and square

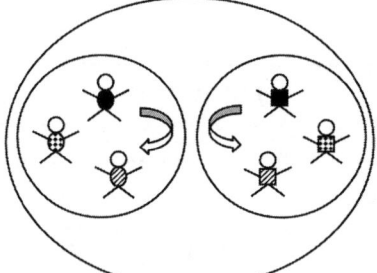

Time 3: In turn, each subgroup explores and
discovers differences within its similarity

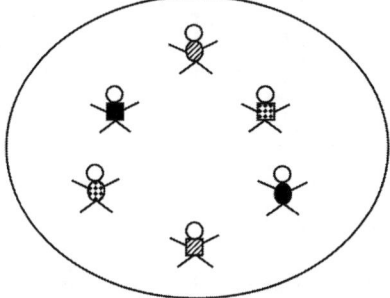

Time 4: Integration in the group-as-a-whole and greater complexity

Figure 1.21

group-as-a-whole. SCT defines this process of discriminating and integrating differences as both a sufficient and necessary condition for group development.

For example, in the new group illustrated in Figure 1.21, group members, as is quite common at the start of a group, are either excited or anxious (Time 1). Using functional subgrouping, those who are anxious talk together and in turn, those who are excited talk to each other (Time 2). Within the security of similarity, the anxious members discover small differences (Time 3): "I feel anxious because I think this is not going to work for me." "My anxiety is coming from how restricted I feel in my body, all uncomfortable." "I'm anxious because I don't know what will happen here." In turn, the excited members explore and find excitement at not knowing, apprehension at not knowing and some discomfort as well as pleasure in their bodies with all the excitement. At this point, the group begins to notice the similarities between the differences and the differences start to integrate. Members then feel more at ease with the differences (Time 4).

Recapping

Returning to our theory statement, a TLHS defines a *hierarchy* of *isomorphic* systems that are *energy-organizing*, *goal-directing* and *self-correcting*. We have now defined the major constructs, hierarchy and isomorphy. We revisit the expanded and illustrated version of our theory chart summarizing the simple definition of *isomorphy* with illustrations that build a bridge from the constructs to the operational definitions (see Figure 1.22).

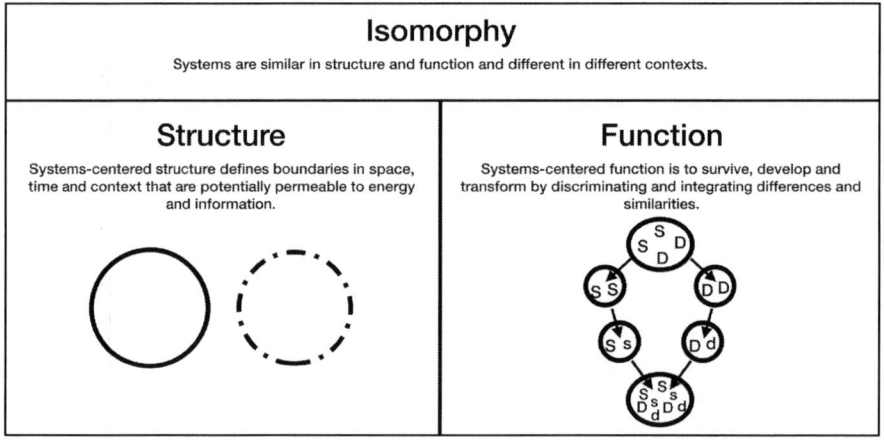

Figure 1.22

We can see quite a bit when looking through the lens of the system's structure and its function. For example, there is an interdependent relationship between the dynamics of structure and function. When the boundary is open to letting in differences (structure), there will be more possibility of discriminating and integrating these differences towards the goal of survival, development and transformation (function). Or when the boundary is closed, the system is more in survival with less potential for development. As isomorphic systems, what is learned about the structure or function of any one system generalizes to every other system in the hierarchy (refer again to Figure 1.8).

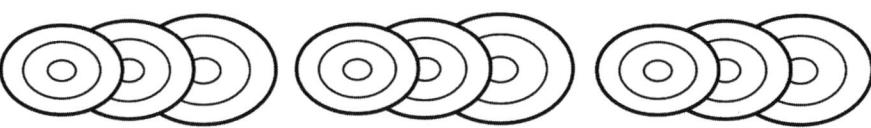

Person - Member - Group   Member - Group - Clinic   Group - Clinic - Hospital

Figure 1.8

By operationally defining isomorphy, methods that are useful to influence structure or function in one system will be useful in all other systems in the hierarchy of living human systems: person, couples, small groups and large and larger and largest groups! For example, functional subgrouping is our method for increasing the probability of discriminating and integrating differences. And with isomorphy, we would expect functional subgrouping to be useful for integrating differences for individuals, couples, groups, organizations and even larger human systems.

Revisiting structure as energy-organizing

SCT systems organize the energy and information that cross system boundaries in the form of "communications" so that the system can use the energy/information and discriminate and integrate it to move towards its goals. The systems-centered structure defines boundaries in space, time and reality that are potentially permeable to energy/information.

Boundaries are defined in time, space and reality

Defining a system in space and time makes an important bridge between ideas and what actually happens in the world. The challenge is to keep making bridges between systems as an abstract idea to real systems in the real world of time and space and reality. A theory is less useful if it does not allow us to see things and do things that we did not see or could not do before we looked at the world through the lens of the theory. Thus, thinking of a group or a person as a system is only an important idea when it can be useful. For example, a group system can only exist in the real world if its members know where and when to meet. If that practical connection is not made, the group system still exists as only an idea, but not in reality. So, if a group is to exist, it must have time boundaries and space boundaries. Why is this a useful thought? When we think of space and time serving as boundaries for the system, we can observe the difference it makes in the ways that group systems function. For example, it makes a difference for how groups function when they stop and start on time and when they don't.

Another practical application of thinking "boundaries" is our past/present/future map (see Figure 1.23) that Yvonne adapted from Lewin (1951b). Each of the six squares in the Cartesian square are separated from each other by a boundary.

Map of Reality and Irreality in the Past, Present and the Future

	Past	Present	Future
Explaining experience (irreality)	Interpreting of memories	Interpreting on the basis of wishes and fears	Making negative and positive predictions
Exploring experience (reality)	Exploring past actions	Exploring present experience Common sense Reality-testing	Making plans and goals

Note. This is an elaboration of Lewin's (1951b) Map of Reality and Irreality in the Past, Present and the Future.

Figure 1.23

In SCT groups, we emphasize exploring in here-and-now reality. Often a group member or several will start telling a story about their past. To cross the boundary from the past to the present, the leader asks: "how is now different from then?" (finding the differences in the apparently similar) (see Figure 1.24).

SCT also emphasizes undoing the positive or negative predictions about the future (the future/irreality square) and crossing the boundary from future irreality to present irreality (see Figure 1.25).

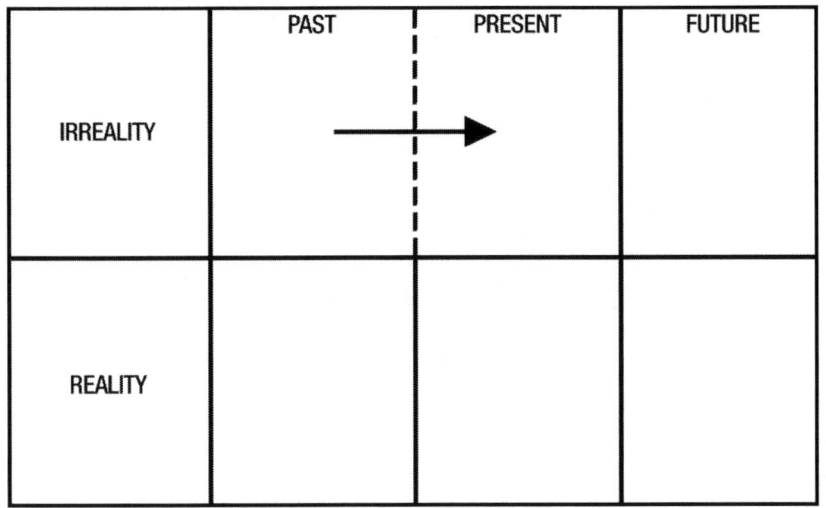

Figure 1.24

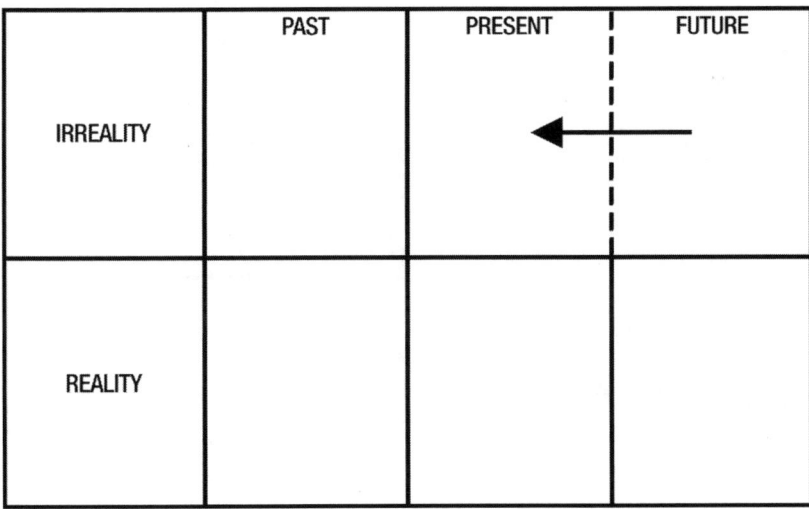

Figure 1.25

In present irreality, group members learn to check their mindreads of others, which starts to build a reality-testing system and crosses the boundary from present irreality to present reality (see Figure 1.26).

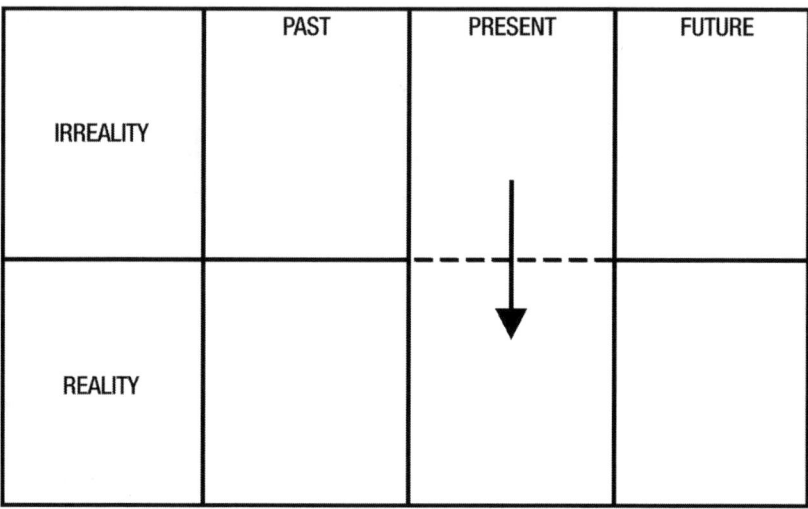

Figure 1.26

By crossing these boundaries, groups learn to shift into present reality (see Figure 1.27).

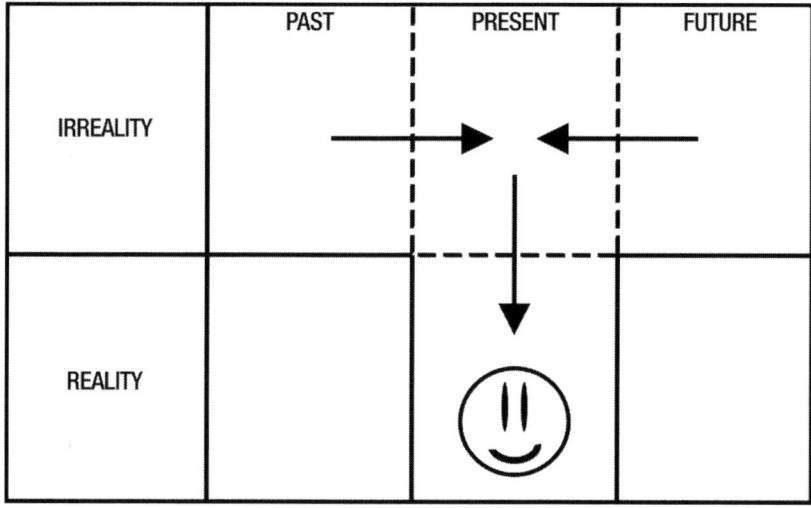

Figure 1.27

In present reality, we can then visit the past for information (cross the boundary from present reality to past reality) and plan for the future (cross the boundary from present reality to future reality plans) (see Figure 1.28).

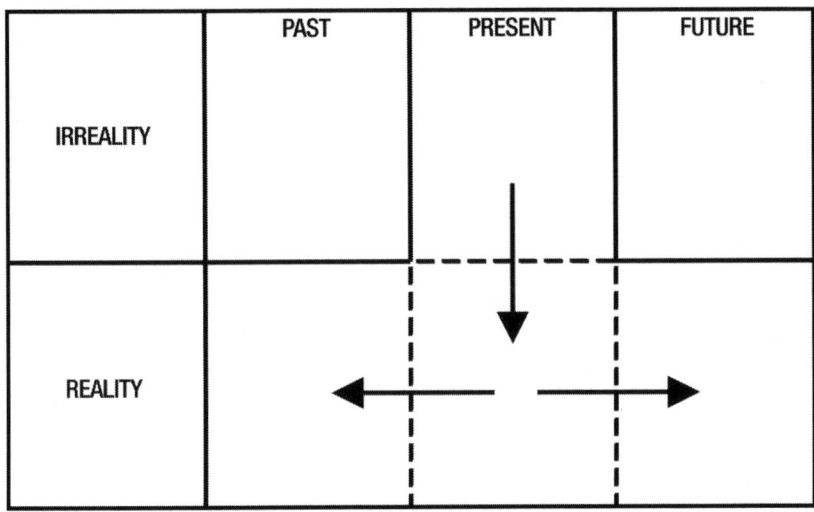

Figure 1.28

Boundaries exist between and within all systems in the hierarchy, circles within circles. These boundaries are potentially permeable to transactions of information and energy. For example, in our past/present/future map (see Figure 1.23), if the boundary is too open from the past to the present, we cannot discriminate easily between present reality and past reality. In theory language, boundaries open or close to the flow of energy/information in the communications across the boundaries of the system hierarchy.

Boundaries open to clear communications and close to noise

We have referred to energy without formally defining it. Succinctly, energy in living human systems is information and the goal of communication in living human systems is the transfer of information across a boundary. This is quite important as living human systems need the information and energy in the differences to develop, so without the transfer of differences, systems can only survive, ultimately becoming entropic. As energy and information are so vital for the survival and development of any living human system, we will revisit this in more depth in the next chapter.

Revisiting hierarchy and its implications for SCT practice

We have now defined isomorphy and how it has been useful in thinking about living human systems. We have also highlighted the methods that operationally define the constructs of structure and function. Next we revisit hierarchy and its operational definition as a set of three nested systems and describe the contextualizing methods that SCT has formulated to apply hierarchy.

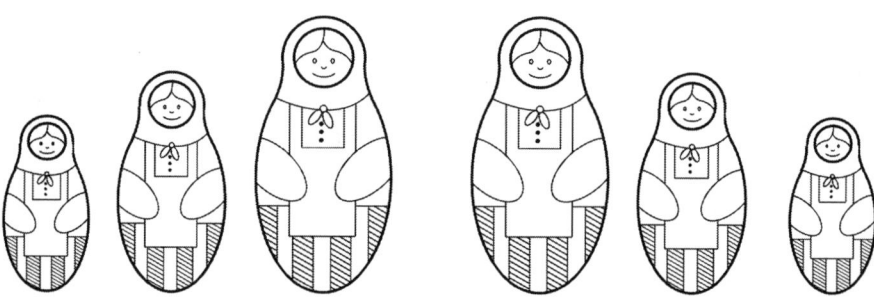

Figure 1.29

We defined hierarchy as systems, from smaller to larger and larger to smaller. Going back to our set of Russian nesting dolls, the middle doll exists in the context of the larger doll and is itself the context for the smaller doll. Every system exists in a context and is a context. In SCT, systems come in threes, and every system is always one of a triad of systems.

Understanding hierarchy has led us to emphasize "context" in our systems-centered therapy and consultation. SCT stresses that as we change contexts (for example from our person system to our member system), our perspective and consequently our experience changes. The perspective from the person system is different from being in a member system, as it is a different context and is different again from experiencing the context of being in a system-as-a-whole like a group. Becoming aware that there are as many different ways of understanding our experience as there are different perspectives reduces the tendency to think that everything (or anything!) is all about us. (The view from the sidewalk is different from the view from the ninth floor, the roof, or an airplane.) The three systems SCT defines are the person system, the member system, the group system-as-a-whole. Member systems form the transitory subsystems, for example, subgroups, that emerge from interactions between members.

Figure 1.30 shows the method of contextualizing which operationally defines hierarchy and puts the theoretical construct into practice.

Contextualizing: activating the observing self-system to perceive the isomorphy in the systems-centered hierarchy.

System-as-a-whole roles: survive, develop and transform within the context of the defined hierarchy.

Subsystem roles: discriminate and integrate information.

Member system roles: direct energy into subsystems.

Person system-as-a-whole: source of primary energy flow.

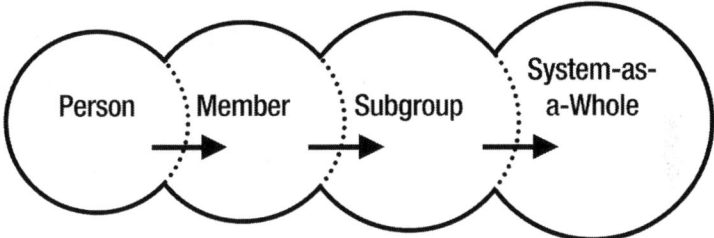

Figure 1.30

Seeing the systems hierarchy

The person system is the center system of the hierarchy and the source of energy for the whole hierarchy.

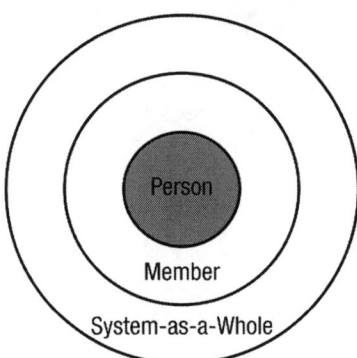

Figure 1.31

It contains the primary energy for survival that not only fuels the person system of an individual but also is the energy that fuels and flows through all living human systems in the hierarchy.

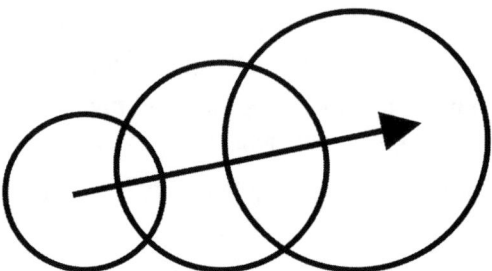

Figure 1.32

The member system is the middle system, and its goal is to develop the system. Within the member system, there are subsystems of member roles and subgroups. Both develop in the middle system and function to discriminate and integrate the similarities and differences, both differences in the apparently similar and similarities in the apparently different.

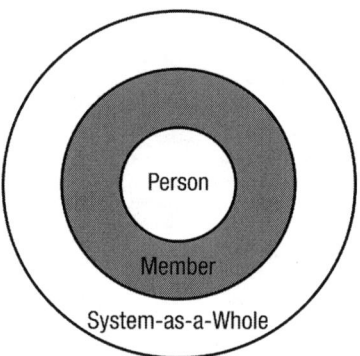

Figure 1.33

The system-as-a-whole is the source of system transformation. This system organizes the discriminations and integrations of energy into system norms. This contains the whole system towards system survival, development and transformation (see Figure 1.34).

When we begin to see a larger context than any one system, we can then perceive the isomorphy beyond a single system (see Figure 1.35). All systems share the same ways that they manage the permeability of their boundaries (structure) and the ways that they function to discriminate and integrate. Thus, what works for any one system works for all systems in the hierarchy!

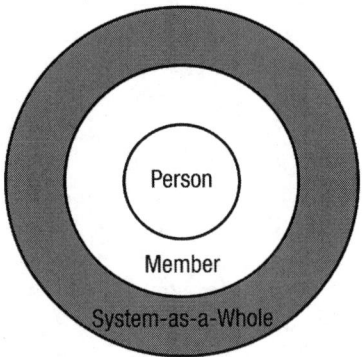

Figure 1.34

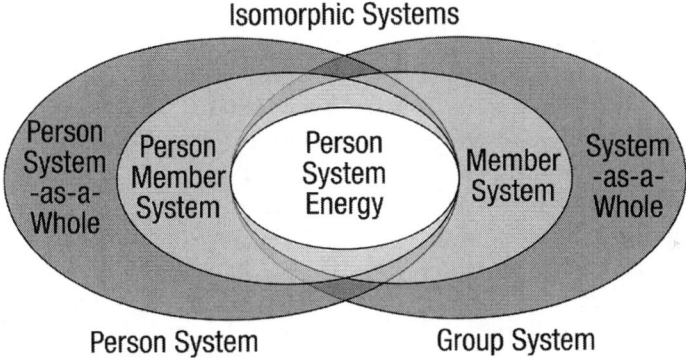

Figure 1.35

The advantage of this illustration is that it lends itself to recognizing the relationship among person, member and system-as-a-whole, not only within the person but also in the whole hierarchy of living human systems, with the person system containing the energy for each transformation.

The SCT hierarchy: implications for psychotherapy, group work and team consultation

The idea that a person can see themselves as three separate but related systems with three separate goals is often a brand-new idea when people first orient themselves to systems-centered theory. It is also one of the most important ideas that systems-centered therapy, training and consultation offers. Seeing ourselves as a triad of systems introduces the reality that there is a difference between experiencing the world as if it is all about us, which SCT calls the personalizing part of our person system, and discovering instead that there are many worlds to be experienced. If we access our curiosity when we cross into our member system and recognize that as a member we relate to outside contexts as well as our personal ones, our experience of the world expands. From our systems perspective we are not one, but three! We have three discrete but related experiences from three separate but interconnected systems! When we become aware of how the three systems are different, we become aware of three different sets of perceptions, three different experiences, and three different perspectives of ourselves and the world around us. The original rationale of presenting them as "separate but interdependent" isomorphic systems was to emphasize that their function changes as the levels in the hierarchy change, as illustrated in Figure 1.35.

Self-centered and systems-centered

Probably the most significant change we make as soon as we see ourselves and the world as systems is that we are less likely to experience the problems that taking things just personally brings. Seeing ourselves and the world through systems eyes gives us a choice between being systems-centered instead of self-centered. The advantage of seeing ourselves as systems-centered is that we have three other perspectives on the world, instead of one. We can see ourselves in the context of being a member in many different contexts: at home, at work and at play. We can see ourselves as being a member of a subgroup, as a compatible (or incompatible) gathering of self and others within different contexts. And (this is a little more unusual) we can see ourselves as existing in subgroups that contribute to building the norms of the system-as-a-whole of which we are a part, that contains subgroups, members and people. Influencing the norms of the systems we live in has the most impact on our freedom to be who we want to be. Taking our role to influence system norms is an ongoing human challenge and is not only the most difficult but also the most important.

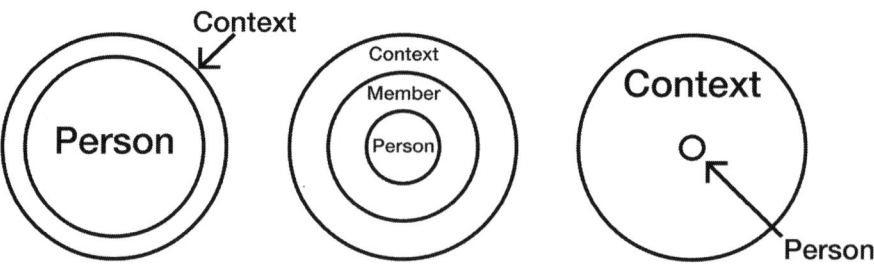

Figure 1.36

Role, goal and context

In SCT, we learn not to take ourselves "just personally." We also learn to see the world through these different systems perspectives and different sets of contexts, each of which contributes to the survival, development and transformation of all living human systems. As we shift from one perspective (e.g., our person system) to another (our member role), our context changes. As we change context, we shift to a different goal. Each time we change context, the goal changes, and we then have the job of changing our member role so that we can contribute to reaching the different goal. This then becomes an ongoing developmental process as we discover a good enough fit between ourselves and the outside world. SCT refers to this as learning to see our role, goal and context wherever we are. It has been a very useful model for not only our patients but also organizations and teams where clarifying role, goal and context is essential to organizational functioning (Gantt, 2005, 2013; Gantt & Agazarian, 2004, 2005, 2007; Solomon-Gillis & Trey, 1997).

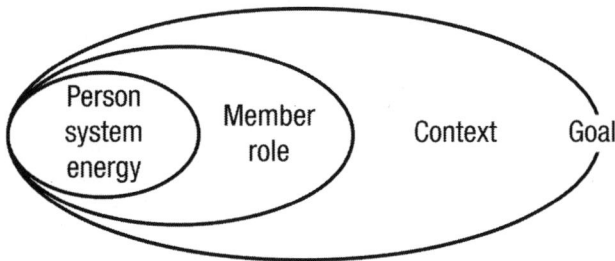

© 2011 Susan Gantt. Adapted from Agazarian, 2012.

Figure 1.37

Our model of role, goal and context puts our triadic system hierarchy into practice. Our three defined systems have important variables in common. Each is fueled by energy. Each has potentially permeable boundaries that allow

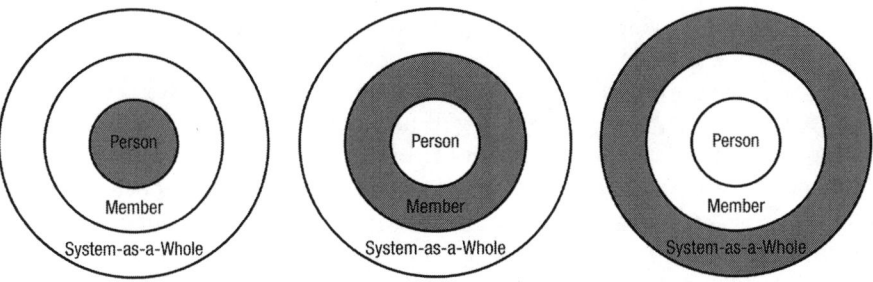

Figure 1.38

exchanges of energy/information to flow between them. Each survives, develops, matures and transforms through discriminating and integrating differences. Each has the potential for developing functional role-systems that interface within and between the different contexts, and each has different goals.

The person system: being me and more

As a person, the context is our self, and our goal is survival and self-development. In contrast, when we become aware of ourselves as a person system, our exploratory drive is re-mobilized and we can solve problems and reach the goals that exist in the present. We become a member of the present context in our self and in our environment. When our context is our self, we can develop our person system. When we become a member of another context, we can take on roles that contribute to the goals of that context.

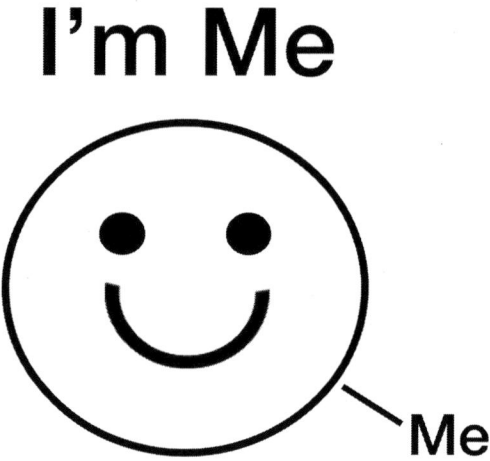

Figure 1.39

In SCT, when someone enters a group, they enter as "a person system." As a person system, the goals are to survive and develop and transform through the influence of the group-as-a-whole. First, however, the person system energy is directed to building the group that will help the group and the people in the group to survive, develop and transform.

It may be a new idea that when we take ourselves just personally, we lose all contexts, even the context of ourselves-as-a-whole. The only system we become aware of then is the system that assumes we are the center of the world and that everything that happens around us is really all about us. When we take things just personally, we are blind to any other perspective and any other context. It is almost impossible to explore reality from a self-centered position. In contrast, when we are in our centered self, we can become aware of ourselves as a "system" with its goal of self-development. It is in our person system that we have the energy for change. It is our person system that will be developed by our member system, subgroup systems and group system-as-a-whole, as we learn to contribute to these specific systems that need to develop to build the group that can develop us!

The member system: learning to be us and we, not just me

As soon as we join a group, we become a member. In SCT, our group member system is different from our person system. As a member system, the goal is to contribute to the development of the group. When members respond to the here-and-now of a group, they develop new roles to solve the group challenges. When members import old roles from the past, they are likely to trigger others to joining them with reciprocal old roles, thus repeating past role relationships into the group. Making this one membership discrimination between past and present has a significant impact on how the membership norms develop in the group. It's quite easy to tell the difference when we or the group do the same thing over and over and when we do something new! This SCT training generalizes to everyday life.

When we as people become members, we have crossed the boundary from our person system into a member system. Whereas the goal of the person system is self-development, the goal of the member system is system development! This idea developed and transformed further in 2014, as will be discussed in the later chapters.

Putting the systems all together

The person system is described as being on the first step on the rung of the ladder of the hierarchy of living human systems. All living human systems are defined as a triad, with a core central system containing the primary energy with the goal of survival, a middle "member" system with the goal of developing through integrating the information from its contexts, the transitory subsystems with the potential to contain and integrate the differences in conflicts, and the system-as-a-whole with the goal of developing the system norms that support the survival, development and transformation of all levels of the hierarchy and which give each system its unique characteristics.

We end this chapter with an excerpt from our theory chart of the theoretical definitions and SCT methods. This chart summarizes the definitions of each construct and, in turn, shows the operational definitions that translate the theory into SCT methods with illustrations of the methods. The complete theory chart which includes the list of techniques that put the methods into practice is included in the appendix of this book.

A THEORY OF LIVING HUMAN SYSTEMS

A theory of living human systems defines a hierarchy of isomorphic systems: energy-organizing, goal-directing and self-correcting.

THEORETICAL DEFINITIONS

HIERARCHY
Systems come in threes. Every system exists in the context of the system above and is the context for the system below.

ISOMORPHY
Systems are similar in structure and function and different in different contexts. There is an interdependent relationship between the dynamics of structure, function and energy at all levels of the systems hierarchy.

CONTEXT
Systems-centered contexts define a recursive triad of isomorphic systems in a defined hierarchy.

STRUCTURE
Systems-centered structure defines boundaries in space, time and context that are potentially permeable to energy / information.

ENERGY
Systems-centered flow of energy and information is defined as a force field of vectors approaching or avoiding system goals.

FUNCTION
Systems-centered function is to survive, develop and transform by discriminating and integrating differences and similarities.

SYSTEMS-CENTERED METHODS

CONTEXT
Contextualizing:
Activating the researcher role to perceive the isomorphy in the systems-centered hierarchy.

System-as-a-whole roles:
Survive, develop and transform within the context of the defined hierarchy.

Member system roles:
Direct energy into subsystems. Discriminate and integrate information.

Person system-as-a-whole:
Source of primary energy / information flow.

STRUCTURE
Boundarying:
Organizing system boundaries.

Survival:
Managing the permeability of system boundaries (in the hierarchy of systems) by reducing noise in the communications within and between all systems and subsystems.

ENERGY
Vectoring:
Directing energy & information flow.

Development:
Directing energy/information towards the primary goals of survival, development and transformation as well as the goals of the context.

FUNCTION
Subgrouping:
Correcting energy & information flow.

Transformation:
Containing, discriminating and integrating differences in the apparently similar and similarities in the apparently different at all system levels.

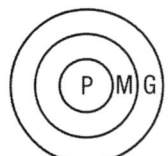
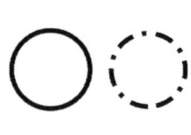
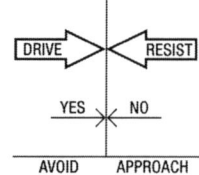
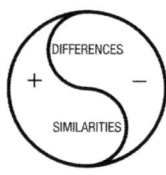

Figure 1.40

The middle column under isomorphy in our excerpt from our theory chart relates to the variable of *goal-directing* and when energy approaches or avoids system goals. We have noted that living human systems are oriented to the primary goals of survival, development and transformation, yet we have not fully discussed the energy which systems structure and function to discriminate and integrate. Energy is fundamental in all living human systems and in system communications within and across boundaries. We will explore more about energy in Chapter 2, where we both present and develop our theoretical formulations of energy and the implications this has had for SCT practice.

References

Agazarian, Y. M. (1997). *Systems-centered therapy for groups*. New York, NY: Guilford Press. Reprinted in paperback (2004). London, UK: Karnac Books.

Bertalanffy, L. V. (1968). *General system theory: Foundations, development, applications* (rev. ed.). New York, NY: George Braziller.

Gantt, S. P. (2005). Functional role-taking in organizations and work groups. *Group Psychologist (APA Division 49 Newsletter)*, *15*(5), 15.

Gantt, S. P. (2013). Applying systems-centered theory (SCT) and methods in organizational contexts: Putting SCT to work. *International Journal of Group Psychotherapy*, *63*(2), 234–258. doi:10.1521/ijgp.2013.63.2.234

Gantt, S. P., & Agazarian, Y. M. (2004). Systems-centered emotional intelligence: Beyond individual systems to organizational systems. *Organizational Analysis*, *12*(2), 147–169. doi:10.1108/eb028990

Gantt, S. P., & Agazarian, Y. M. (Eds.). (2005). *SCT in action: Applying the systems-centered approach in organizations*. Lincoln, NE: iUniverse. Reprint (2006). London, UK: Karnac Books.

Gantt, S. P., & Agazarian, Y. M. (2007). Phases of system development in organizational work groups: The systems-centered approach for intervening in context. *Organisational & Social Dynamics*, *7*(2), 253–291.

Lewin, K. (1951a). Problems of research in social psychology. In D. Cartwright (Ed.), *Field theory in social science: Selected theoretical papers* (pp. 155–169). New York, NY: Harper & Row.

Lewin, K. (1951b). *Field theory in social science*. New York, NY: Harper & Row.

Solomon-Gillis, C., & Trey, B. (1997). Applying systems-centered theory (SCT) to organizational consulting. *SCT Journal: Systems-Centered Theory and Practice*, *2*, 39–42.

Chapter 2

Energy, information and communication

From the beginning of time, human beings have wondered where life comes from, what energy is and how energy gives life. Over the years, we have discovered and developed many different and similar systems of thought to answer these questions. For SCT, we have considered how life force energy might be derived from the cosmic, universal energy of the universe, which organizes to form planets like our own where life has evolved in its many forms. We have equated the life force energy with this universal, existential energy. The life force contains the drive to survive, develop and transform from simpler to more complex in all living human systems.

One of the major goals in SCT is to develop the capacity for common sense in everyday life, which starts by first becoming aware of the life force in ourselves as the source of energy for personal survival, development and change.

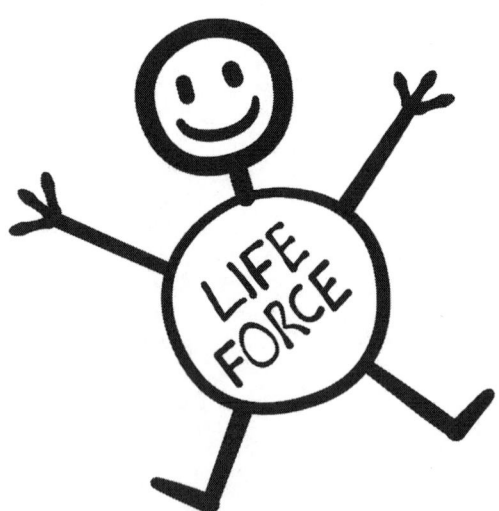

Figure 2.1

Experiencing our awareness of the life force allows us to see that the boundaries of our evolution are permeable to the energy of the universe. Some of us experience a sense that we are somehow one with the universe on the one hand as well as one with the existential energy of ourselves on the other. Experiencing our energy connects us to the universe and all energy and matter in it. It also connects us to each other with the experience of energy between us.

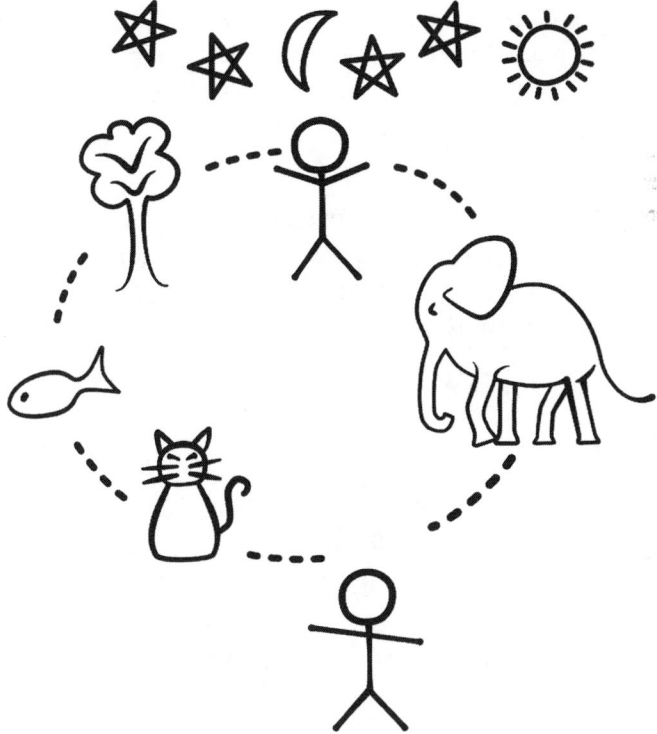

Figure 2.2

The universal, existential energy is the life force fuel for all living human systems and all human hierarchies of living systems. How this system energy is organized, directed and integrated impacts how the system functions on the path to the primary goals of survival, development and transformation and the secondary goal of environmental mastery. SCT specifies the secondary goal as work (Agazarian, 1997), for example, towards the goals of therapy, family life, a partnership, the workplace or any living human system.

In contrast to using our energy for development and work, our energy can be organized only for survival. For example, when our energy is dominated by negative predictions based on past experience, it becomes difficult to take in any new reality data in the present that could impact our present and our future. Without addressing this, we are bound to repeat old patterns of behavior that were developed to manage an old situation. Similarly, when energy about our physiological experience of the present is bound up or "straightjacketed" in tension, we lose access to our energy as a valuable resource for our development. The same is true of depression and outrage, where the vital energy and information in anger, passion, aggression and the retaliatory impulse is either vectored towards our self as the target or discharged in the environment in outrage and acting out. In either case, the energy and information are unavailable for development or work.

SCT defines two forms of energy

SCT has also discriminated two kinds of energy in living human systems. First is the existential life force energy in the core energy system (the center circle in our triad), with its primary goal of survival. The second is the energy to explore that can cross the boundaries between the core energy system and its context and has the goal of development.

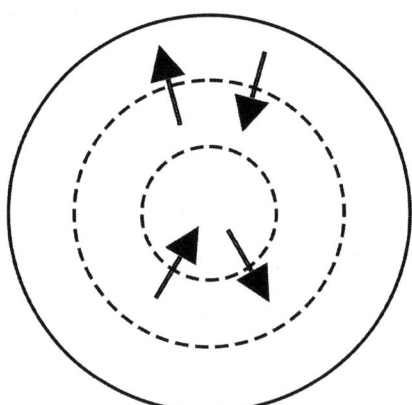

Figure 2.3

How these energies travel through a system and its hierarchy of systems will have an impact on the system reaching its primary goals of survival, development and transformation as well as the secondary goals that are the stated goals of the system. As human beings, we are born with existential energy as well as the energy which leads us to find out about the world inside us and around us. It is in directing our energies through our curiosity that we come to understand how we survive, develop and transform ourselves at each stage of our lives – from infant to toddler to student to adult to senior.

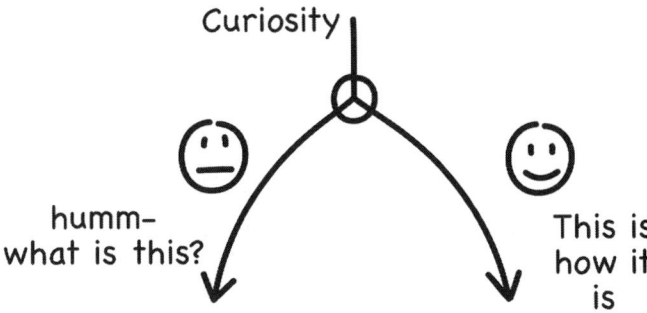

Figure 2.4

Communication and communication vectors

SCT (Agazarian, 1997) borrowed the idea of equating energy with information from physics (Miller, 1978). Equating energy and information in living human systems, communication can then be defined as the transfer of energy/information (E/I) across system boundaries.

Shannon and Weaver (1964), in their book *The Mathematical Theory of Communication*, demonstrated that ambiguities and redundancy are entropic noise in the communication channel. Their mathematical formulas showed that the more noise in the communication channel, the less likely it is that the information in the communication will get across. Later, we added contradictions as a third source of noise or entropic communication (Simon & Agazarian, 1967, 2000). This understanding of noise helped us formulate communication as a vector that transfers energy and information across a boundary. This then led us to use an arrow to depict vectors of energy and information.

The arrow

The arrow has been almost as important as the circle in working out our theory. When we talk about energy and transferring energy, we can represent it in the image of an arrow that carries the energy and information and moves in a direction.

We use the arrow to illustrate the movement of energy.

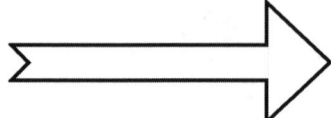

Figure 2.5

By definition, an arrow moves in a direction.

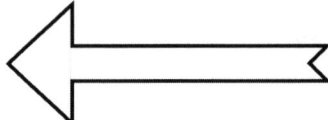

Figure 2.6

Arrows can move in any direction, any which way.

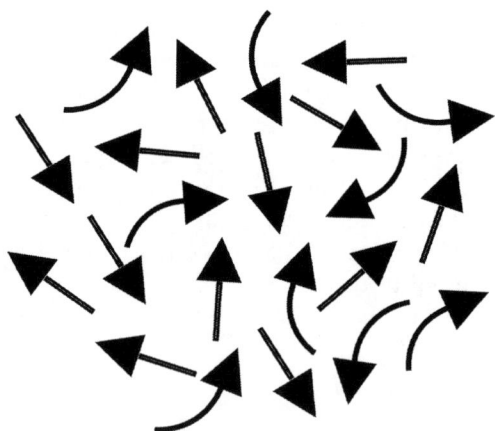

Figure 2.7

The arrow carries the system energy.

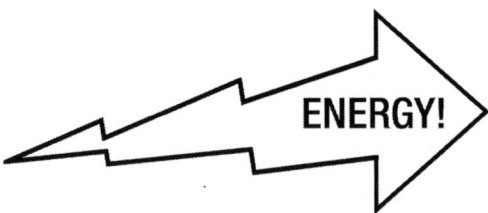

Figure 2.8

We call the arrow that carries the system energy in a direction a vector.

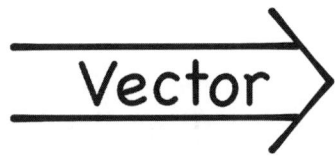

Figure 2.9

The arrow or vector carries energy and information; as we said, energy = information (E/I) and information = energy (I/E).

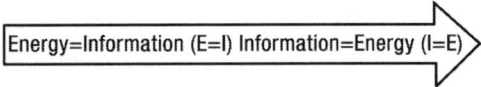

Figure 2.10

In equating energy and information, we have built a bridge between the abstract idea of systems and the practical idea of communication which can be observed and tested to see whether the communication works (Agazarian, 1997).

The E/I is transferred in the form of communication and carried in a communication vector.

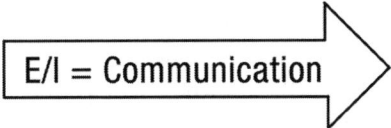

Figure 2.11

It is common sense for many of us that we transfer information when we communicate.

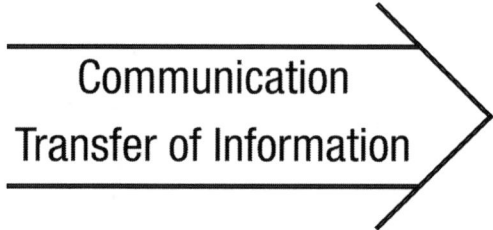

Figure 2.12

However, it is unusual and important to think of the transfer of information as the transfer of energy. We build on this idea by calling the vectors that carry energy/information "communication vectors."

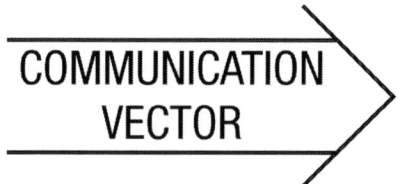

Figure 2.13

Communication vectors

The goal of communication is to transfer the energy/information. For example, if I tell you how I feel, the goal of my communication is to transfer the information in my feelings to you so that you know how I feel too. Or the communication can be from me to me: I know I am getting anxious but I don't know why. Connecting to myself more fully allows me to know what I know about the source of my anxiety. This is a transfer of energy/information from the part of me who knows to the part of me who doesn't know.

Communication vectors contain the energy/information that crosses the boundaries in living human systems and, by so doing, provide the energy

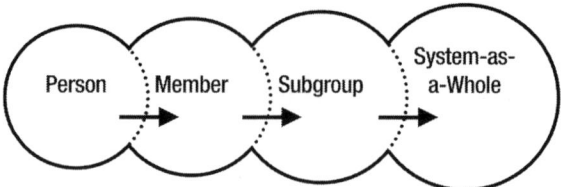

Figure 2.14

and information that all systems require if they are to survive, develop and transform.

Communication is the transfer of energy/information across the boundaries between and within systems in the hierarchy.

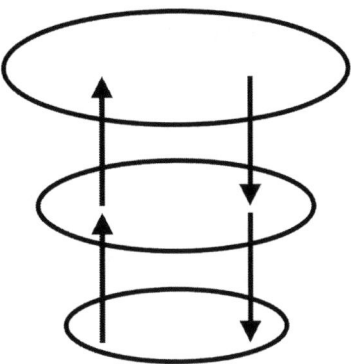

Figure 2.15

Returning to Shannon and Weaver (1964), we can also say that in a communication vector, there is always both noise and information.

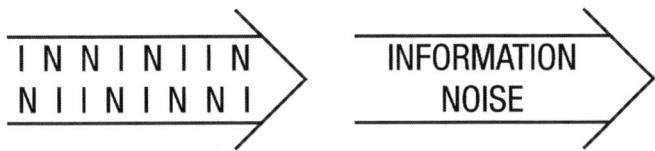

Figure 2.16

The degree of noise in the communication predicts the potential for energy/information to get across the boundary from one system to another. The more noise in the vector, the less information is transferred. Or we could say, in noisy communications, very little information crosses the boundary. The amount of energy/information that is transferred across the boundary then influences how much energy is available for development. For example, if the information is packaged in an attacking communication (note: "attacking" is noise in a communication vector), the receiving system is likely to defend by either attacking back, defending oneself, attacking oneself (also noise) or leaving. In any case, it is unlikely the actual information could be used for development or problem-solving.

When communication vectors contain more information than noise, they are more likely to successfully convey information across the boundary into the system.

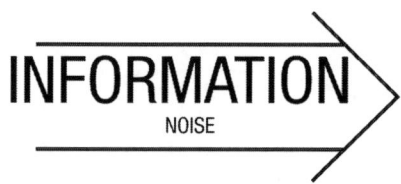

Figure 2.17

When communication vectors contain more noise than information, very little information will cross the boundary. Systems tend to close their boundaries to noise. When this happens, communication vectors are blocked at the boundary.

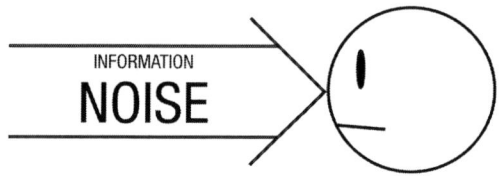

Figure 2.18

This work with understanding communication as the transfer of energy/ information in a communication vector that crosses the boundary has helped us deepen our understanding of the process of discriminating and integrating differences that is so central to development in living human systems.

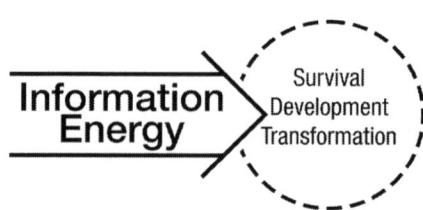

Figure 2.19

Discriminating and integrating differences

As we discussed in Chapter 1, discriminating and integrating differences fuels development. All energy and information will contain similarities and differences. For a system to develop, it has to open its boundary to energy/information to take in differences that can be discriminated and integrated.

Similar enough

If the energy/information is similar enough to what we already know or feel, we can take it in easily.

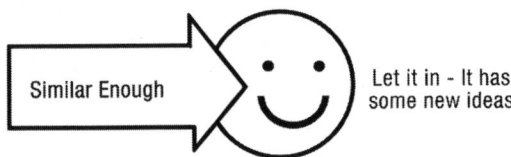

Figure 2.20

Too much similarity: redundant noise

On the other hand, when too much similarity enters the system, it introduces noise in the form of redundancy. Redundancy fixates a system in what it already knows. Redundancy in the communication vector interferes with the transfer of energy/information that is necessary for development. For example, when someone is trying to say something and they repeat the same thing over and over (redundancy), it is likely we will stop listening ("not again!") and tune out or get bored. In a therapy group, we can also see this when the group repeats the same communication pattern among members or is stuck talking about the same thing over and over. Too much similarity is also a problem if there is not enough difference to activate the discrimination and integration necessary for development.

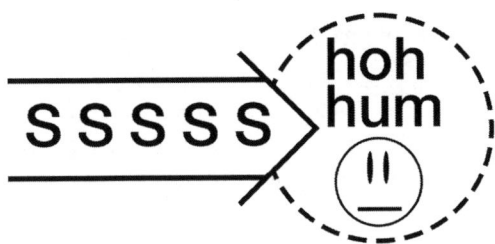

Figure 2.21

Too much difference

On the other hand, when there is too much difference or contradiction entering the system, it introduces another kind of noise.

When too much difference enters the system, the system is under threat of de-differentiation where more energy comes in than the system can organize and use, often leading to internal disorganization and chaos.

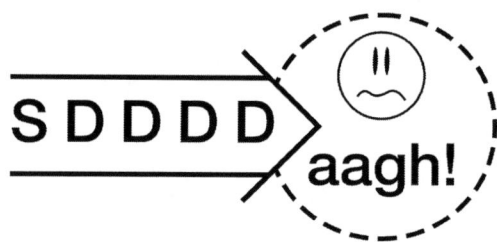

Figure 2.22

To manage "too much" difference, the system may encapsulate the differences in a containing subsystem. Groups often close boundaries to "too much" difference by creating an identified patient or scapegoat role. Sometimes these "too different" differences are encapsulated in closed boundaried subsystems in oneself, common with trauma.

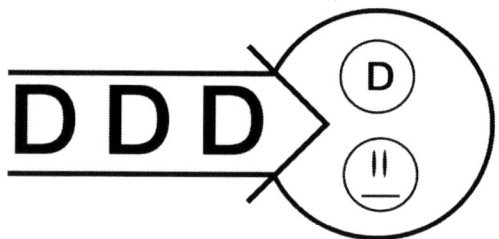

Figure 2.23

More implications from seeing communication vectors

The idea that communication vectors transfer energy and information has important implications for listening to what people say in groups and how they say it. It influences how SCT therapists listen to the flow of words in groups. On the one hand, SCT therapists attune to the information in the content and the meaning this information has for the patient in their system roles of person and member. On the other hand, the SCT therapists pay attention to how much energy is available for work in the group by tracking closed and open boundaries.

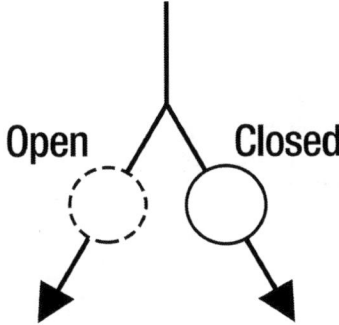

Figure 2.24

An additional advantage of thinking about the direction that the group is moving in terms of the communication vectors is that the therapist can help the group re-vector away from resistances. For example, a re-vectoring intervention to a group that is moving towards flight is to ask, "what is the goal of the group at this moment?" Another example in a group that is eliciting an identified patient role is to ask whether it would be useful to the group to explore the two sides of trying to "take care of" a member in the group, testing to see whether there is a subgroup with the impulse to "cure" the patient and another subgroup with the impulse to "get rid of" the person in the role. Both these interventions encourage members to discover vectors that they were unaware they had and introduce them to a familiarity with two systems: the known and the not-yet-known.[1]

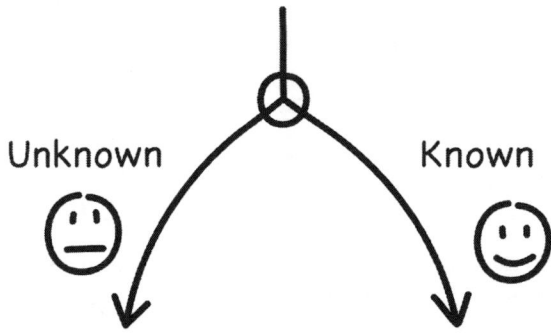

Figure 2.25

When therapists or consultants orient themselves to the energy flow in the group, there are many questions to ask: In what direction is the energy flowing in the group?

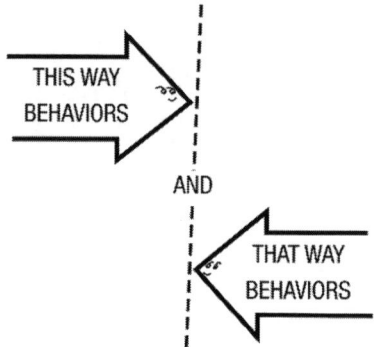

Figure 2.26

Is the energy organized into explaining with mindreads and negative predictions? Is the energy bound up in tension? Is the energy free for exploration or blocked in explanations?

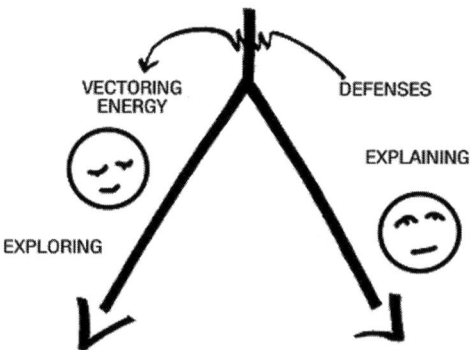

Figure 2.27

Is the energy vectored into depression or discharged in outrage? Are members joining one another or fighting over differences? Is the energy directing the group from one phase of development towards the next? Can the group's direction be interpreted as flight energy from the conflicts within a phase? Is the group energy moving towards expressing its frustrations in a fight? Has it solved its phase conflict by vectoring its energy into a premature intimacy? When there is silence, is the energy in the silence a contemplative one? Is it a pause while the group makes a transition from one level of understanding to another? Or is it a sulky silence where the group seems dead in the water? ("Dead in the water" is often a signal that the group is having an unspoken conflict with the therapist.)

Adapting Lewin's force field

In asking these questions about energy flow, we adapted Lewin's (1951) model of the force field to collect and organize information about communication. Lewin introduced the force field as a way to map the equilibrium of driving and restraining forces moving towards or away from a goal.

By collecting the information in a force field, we can then see whether the communication vector is moving towards the goal of transferring information or towards a different goal. Again, using Lewin's work, we call these vectors driving and restraining forces. By charting the driving and restraining communication vectors, we can learn something about both what the group says it has come together to do (explicit goal) and what it actually is doing that is implied by the communication behavior (the implicit goal). For example, if a couple comes to a therapy session with the explicit goal of working on their relationship and uses the verbal behavior of attack/blame/self-defense (noise), we can infer that the implicit goal of the couple's system is to fight (see Figure 2.28).

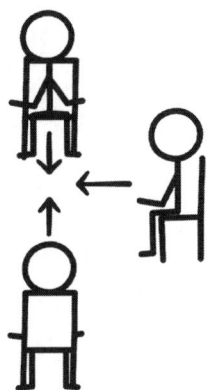

Figure 2.28

Or, when we as therapists ask a question or reflect a client and are met with a "yes, but," we can infer that the boundary is closed to input from us as we have likely introduced a difference that was too different.

Here is a force field of communication vectors (see Figure 2.29). The restraining forces listed are the three kinds of noise in a communication vector, drawing from Shannon and Weaver (1964) and Simon and Agazarian (1967, 2000). These noisy behaviors move towards an implicit goal of avoiding information transfer. In contrast, the driving forces would contribute to clear communication.

Communication Vectors	
Driving ⟹	⟸ Restraining
Clear Communication	Noisy Communication
Specificity ⟹	⟸ Ambiguous
Build on Others ⟹	⟸ Contradicts
Concise ⟹	⟸ Redundant
Explicit Goal ⟹	⟸ Implicit Goal

Figure 2.29

Driving and restraining forces in communication vectors

Translating these ideas into practice, we discovered how to reduce "yes, buts" (contradictions), vagueness (ambiguity) and repetitive language (redundancy) in communications. This led to increased understanding but also to an improved climate. Members understood each other and themselves more easily. This was a good example where theory helped us to put some useful methods into practice.[2]

This is also why one of the first things that SCT now does in all groups is reduce the ambiguity, redundancy, and also the contradictions that are concealed in "yes, but" language. With too much noise, the information in the communication tends to get lost in the reactions to the manner of delivery. This of course is true for all systems and all forms of verbal output – thinking, speaking and even for written communication like emails.

From the very beginning of her work, Yvonne has emphasized paying attention to noise in relationship to the context and the goal. For example, in new SCT groups, leaders immediately focus on weakening the noisy communications so that the group can communicate! The first "noise" that is modified are the social communications which in a therapy or training group are restraining forces which block authentic communication. Yet in the context of social situations, social communication is quite driving, as it tends to smooth the way in social situations where the goal is socializing. In the context of a therapy group, however, the therapeutic goals require exploring conflicts rather than smoothing them over. Any behavior or communication can be driving or restraining depending on the goal and context.

More on using the force field to track energy

In the figures that follow, we can see how lying down is a driving force for sleeping, yet it is a restraining force if we are sleeping on the job. Sitting down can be a driving force when the goal is to wait in a waiting room and a restraining force when the goal is to go shopping for dinner. Can you think of a driving *and* restraining force for the figure watching TV and the figure running?

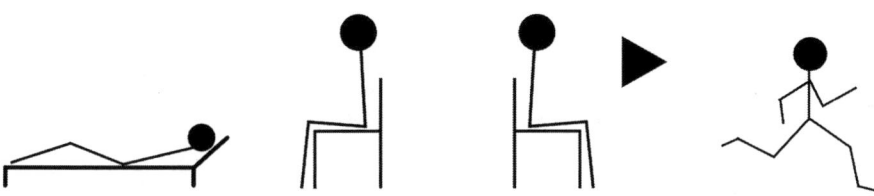

Figure 2.30

Vectors in a force field identify the driving and restraining forces in relationship to the system goals. The force field can then be used to determine where the system is located on its path to the goal.

In Figure 2.31 (Agazarian, 1992, p. 194), we have expanded and elaborated the force field that illustrates the relationship between clear communication (driving forces when the goal is communication) and noisy communication (restraining forces to communication).

Communication Vectors in a Force Field

Force field of driving and restraining forces in
influencing boundary permeability to communication

Driving forces $\rightarrow$	$\leftarrow$	Restraining forces	
(Deduce the explicit goal)		(Deduce the implicit goal)	
Asking direct questions $\rightarrow$	$\leftarrow$	Indirect questions	
	$\leftarrow$	Leading and sarcastic questions	
Answering questions $\rightarrow$	$\leftarrow$	Avoiding answering	
	$\leftarrow$	Changing the subject	
	$\leftarrow$	Answering a question with a question	
Building on ideas $\rightarrow$	$\leftarrow$	Preempting ideas	
	$\leftarrow$	Yes, butting	
	$\leftarrow$	Interrupting	
Supporting oneself and others $\rightarrow$	$\leftarrow$	Putting self or others down	
Proposing $\rightarrow$	$\leftarrow$	Should, "Well everyone knows"	
Owning own feelings $\rightarrow$	$\leftarrow$	Blaming and complaining	
Goal:		Goal:	
Opening boundaries to $\rightarrow$	$\leftarrow$	Closing boundaries to	
Communication and		Communication and	
Energy/Information Flow		Energy/Information Flow	

Figure 2.31

We have also found that the force field is particularly helpful in identifying the range of restraining forces so that we can assess which restraining forces would be the easiest to modify in the communication to make it more likely that the message will get across. All systems in a hierarchy of systems are similar in both their function and in their structure (whether the system is a person, a subgroup or an organization). This enables us to see that the interventions that work to reduce noise in any one system will also work to reduce the noise in all other systems.

Energy in our hierarchy of systems

As we have noted, the energy throughout the hierarchy of systems is fueled by the center system. However, for energy to move from one system to another throughout the hierarchy, it needs to be organized into vectors.

Energy entering from the middle system (member and subgroup) is organized into subsystems that are a resource for the transformation of the system-as-a-whole (see Figure 2.32). The system-as-a-whole has the goal of transformation and system norms and also has the potential for sending the energy/information in a communication across the boundary and taking up a "member" role in the system above it. Thus, subsystems communicate initially (represented by arrows) from the system below each system to the system above each system. We can trace the relationship between middle system subsystems and the transfer of energy and resources throughout the hierarchy.

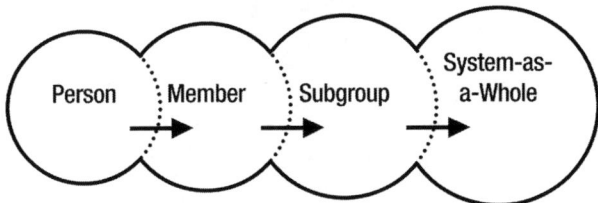

Figure 2.32

The center circle has the goal of survival which is necessary for development, and development is necessary for transformation (see Figure 2.33). The center core system is the source of system energy: the life force that flows throughout the hierarchy.

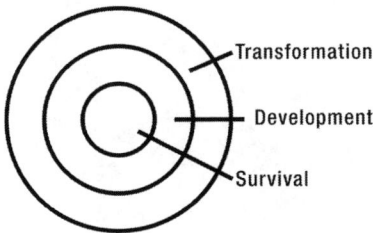

Figure 2.33

The core system: person system

The person system driving forces organize energy to cross the boundaries inside oneself (survival) and, in turn, to cross the boundaries to outside system contexts of member, subgroup and group-as-a-whole. At the same time, the person restraining forces are closed system boundaries to energy inside one-self, taking things "just" personally or closed boundaries to information from outside contexts. When the person system is dominated by the subsystem that takes things just personally, the boundary is closed to all the other subsystems within the person (like roles or clusters of roles in subgroups). When taking things just personally, we are unable to cross the boundaries into the outside system contexts of the member, subgroup or group-as-a-whole and we are unable to take in useful resources from these systems.

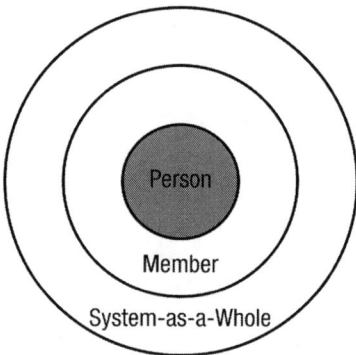

Figure 2.34

Middle system: the member system

The middle member system organizes energy from the person system and is the source of system development. The member system functions to discriminate and integrate energy/information. It is the energy/information in our subsystem roles that give us our resources for managing the various systems of which we are a part in everyday life.

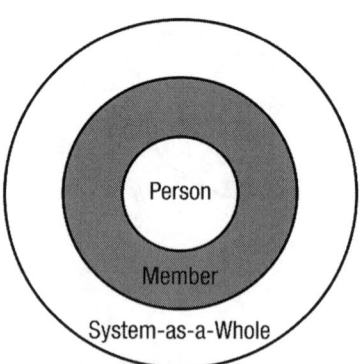

Figure 2.35

The driving forces at this system level are developing functional role-systems related to the goals of the present context. The boundaries open to exploratory energy and functional role relationships. The balancing restraining forces import old role-systems from the past and out of context that repeat the known at the expense of problem-solving in the present.

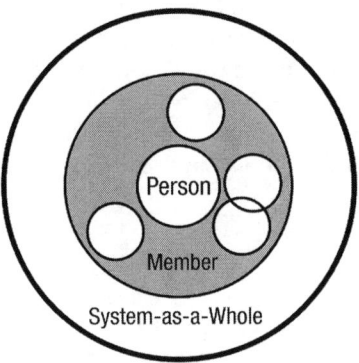

Figure 2.36

Outer system: system-as-whole

The outer system functions to organize the energy of system transformation by integrating the information in the subsystems that develop in the middle system. The major restraining forces within the system-as-a-whole arise from the conflict between the work of developing norms that potentiate a transforming culture (driving force) and the inevitable restraining forces that inhibit the development within each phase.

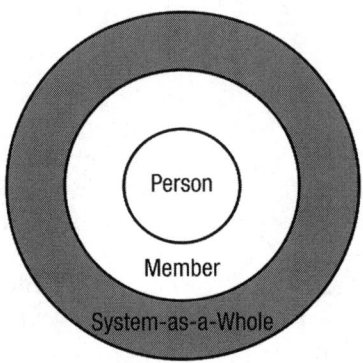

Figure 2.37

Goal-directing

In the previous chapter we focused on structure (energy-organizing) and function (self-correcting). In this chapter, we have shifted our focus to energy which relates to the variable of goal-directing. In SCT, the flow of energy and information is defined as a force field of vectors approaching or avoiding system goals. Just as the clarity of boundaries (structure) influences group energy, the ability of the group to use its energy to reach its goals is determined by how clear the goals are and how surely they are kept in focus.

System energy is always directed towards or away from its goals. The primary goals for all living human systems are to survive, develop and transform, from simpler systems to more complex systems. Goals determine the behavior of the group-as-a-whole and its subgroups. Every group has both a primary and secondary goal.

Primary goals

Primary goals are internal system goals that relate to the survival and development of any living human system. For example, in a group, as the group develops, it transforms from simpler to complex. All living human systems have the inherent driving force towards the primary goals of survival, development and transformation. Helping the group to maintain its boundaries (in space and time) and facilitating clear communications across the boundaries gives the group useful guidelines for its primary goals, survival and development and transformation.

Secondary goals

Secondary goals are the external system goals that relate to solving the problems in mastering its environment. Secondary goals relate to the goal the group was organized to do. A major driving force towards reaching secondary goals is to remind the group what its goal is.

Explicit and implicit goals

Earlier we introduced the idea of explicit and implicit goals. Primary and secondary goals can each be either explicit (acknowledged as the stated purpose of the group) or implicit (the goal the group is behaving "as if" it has), and the explicit and implicit goals can be congruent or incongruent with each other. If the group is behaving in a certain way implicitly because of conflicts with the group's primary or secondary goal (or both), the only energy the group will have available for its work will be whatever energy is free from its conflict. Every system (the subgroup and member and group-as-a-whole) in a group must solve the problems in development that lie on the path to their external goals.

Restraining forces

In SCT, we have built on Lewin's (1951) findings that it is easier to reduce the restraining forces in the way of a goal than it is to increase the driving forces. Maintaining a system's goal direction is achieved by reducing the restraining forces that lie in its way on its path towards its goal, which then releases the driving forces towards the goal. Theoretically then, all living human systems can change course in relationship to their goals by weakening the restraining forces and increasing goal clarity. In practice, this is achieved by influencing the balance of driving and restraining forces in the context of the phase of system development.

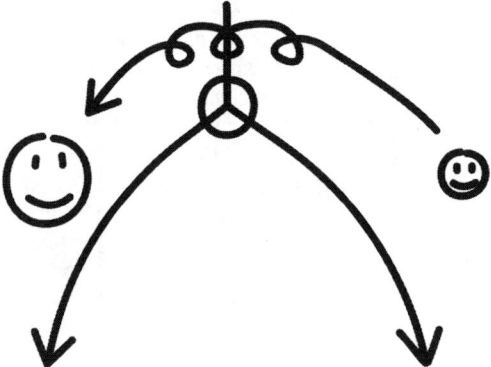

Figure 2.38

When restraining forces are reduced, the drive energy is free to move the system along the path to its goals. For example, if we are trying to go through a closed door, we can run into it with more and more energy until we finally break it down or we can simply open the door that is restraining our entry to the next room. At another time, it might be a driving force to use all that energy against the door to keep someone out.

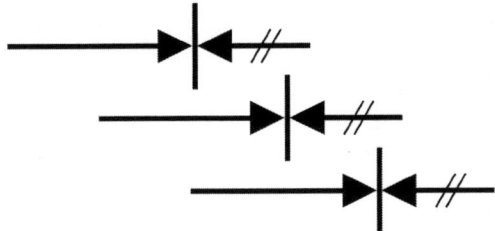

Figure 2.39

The balance between the driving and restraining vectors determines the strength of the drives as well as the probability that information will be transferred. This balance or equilibrium also enables us to diagnose the location of the system in relation to its goals. When we know this, we can see which restraining forces would be easiest to reduce to free the developmental energy in the driving forces without destabilizing the system too much.

Returning to system function and the interdependence of structure, energy and function

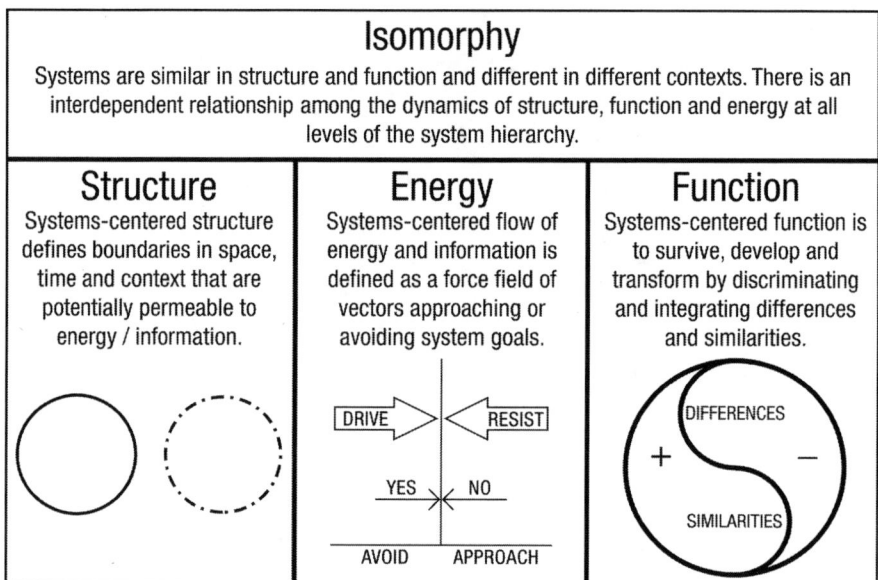

Figure 2.40

The challenges for living human systems in integrating differences occur in all the different groups that we human beings form, and these challenges can have big consequences. Our acute awareness of our human tendency to attack differences by trying to convert them, institutionalize them, ostracize them, persecute them or go to war with them was a major motivation in our development of the systems-centered approach.

Systems develop by integrating energy/information: recognizing what is different in what seemed to be similar and recognizing what is similar in what seemed to be different. This increases both the range of information that systems integrate and the system complexity. When systems integrate new information, the system itself not only develops increased complexity but also develops in its capacity to discriminate and integrate more and more complex information. This is just like a human cell that starts as a single cell and develops from that single cell into a complex, multifunctional organism of cells.

We have discussed how noise in communication vectors both influences boundary permeability and lowers the likelihood of successful communication. We have also talked about how the energy of differences is essential for development. Yet differences when they are "too different" are contradictions (noise) which close a system's boundaries or disrupt its internal organization of energy. For example, a "yes, but" contradiction signals a difference that is "too different." When differences are "too different" from the organization of information within the system, the system reacts to the difference that is too different as contradictory noise and closes its boundaries.

Revisiting functional subgrouping with our eye on energy

Through the lens of energy and communication, functional subgrouping is a method for working with energy so that the group can integrate the similarities and differences in energy/information.

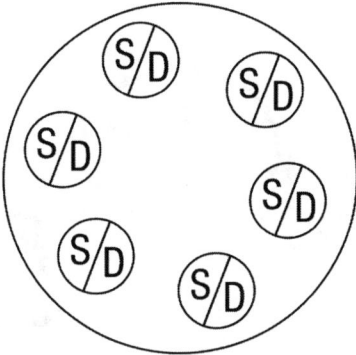

Figure 2.41

Our method of functional subgrouping has enabled us to discriminate and integrate differences and similarities as an alternative to creating identified patients and scapegoats. In a systems-centered group, when differences that are too different to be easily integrated arise, another subgroup is formed to contain and explore the differences and the similarities within the difference. By separating the "too different" differences into different subgroups, potentially alienating differences are contained without disruption to the group system-as-a-whole and can, as they are explored, become a resource for the system.

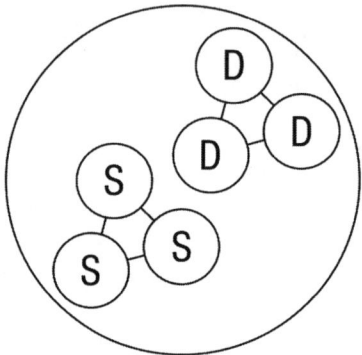

Figure 2.42

These "containing" subgroups have similar energy/information in themselves, but different energy from the other subgroups. Within the comfortable similarity in each subgroup, small differences are safely surfaced and integrated. As subgroup systems integrate small differences, both the subgroup and the system-as-a-whole increase their capacity to discriminate and integrate bigger differences.

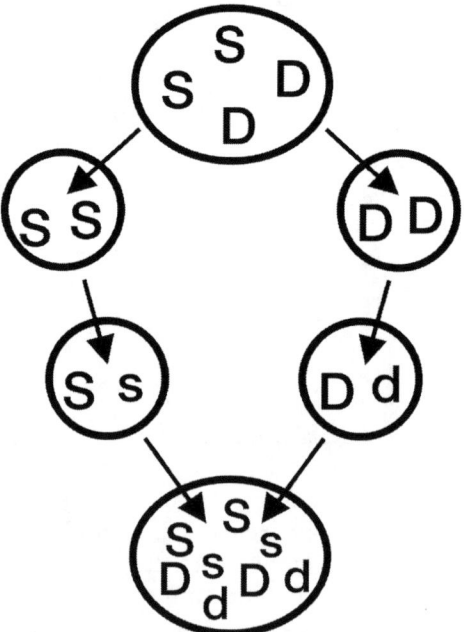

Figure 2.43

As the capacity and range of difference increases within each subgroup, there comes a moment in time when each subgroup recognizes the similarities in what had been apparently different between the two subgroups. At this point, a new integration takes place in the group system-as-a-whole. The group has not only increased its capacity to discriminate and integrate differences, it has also increased in complexity and has more differences available to use as resources.

Joining a subgroup with similarities

Putting together our earlier work on energy crossing the boundary, we can think about how subgroup systems open and close their boundaries. Subgroups integrate differences easily when the energy/information is similar enough to the organizations of information that already exist in the subgroup. These are the "just noticeable differences" in the subgroup system that give us little trouble (see Figure 2.44).

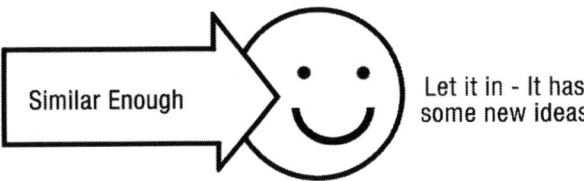

Figure 2.44

Functional subgrouping lowers the tendency to see differences as too different and contradictory, as subgrouping requires joining on a similarity first before adding small differences. Integration is relatively easy when members build on each other in similar enough resonance with both the emotion and content of the message within a supportive subgroup.

Subgroups close their boundaries to communications that are too different

When information is too different, it introduces noise and threatens to disorganize the subgroup system. Often subgroup systems close their boundaries to information that is too different and disruptive to their internal organization. In SCT, instead of just closing off to the difference, we form a new subgroup in the group to explore the difference. Figure 2.45 shows the signal that it is time for a new subgroup to form as the difference is too different for the existing one.

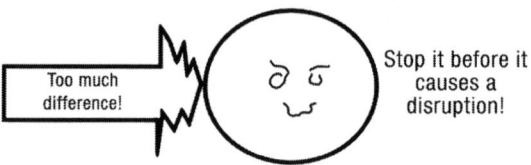

Figure 2.45

To reiterate, the advantage of functional subgrouping in systems-centered groups is that the group system-as-a-whole can contain differences in energy by splitting the "too different" between different subgroups. As each subgroup discriminates and integrates small differences in their subgroup of similarity, each subgroup develops an increased capacity to discriminate and integrate larger differences. As the capacity to integrate differences increases in each of the containing subgroups, there comes a point in time when similarities are recognized between the so-called "different" subgroups and integration then takes place in the group system-as-a-whole.

Monitoring the subgrouping

Sometimes, however, the subgroup boundaries fail to close to "too different" differences. When a difference tries to join the subgroup and the subgroup does not say "stop, that is too different," the internal organization of the subgroup is disrupted and threatened by chaos (see Figure 2.46).

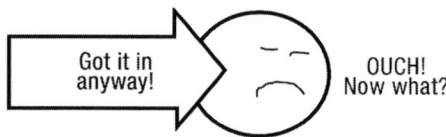

Figure 2.46

Systems-centered therapists are alert for these subgroup failures, as they almost always signal differences that have not been clearly surfaced as a separate subgroup. In addition, SCT leaders monitor when information being added to the subgrouping becomes too similar to the existing organization of the subgroup system and the work becomes redundant. Redundancy creates noise. With redundancy, nothing changes and not only is the information not used in the service of system development but it also fixates development and may even threaten system survival.

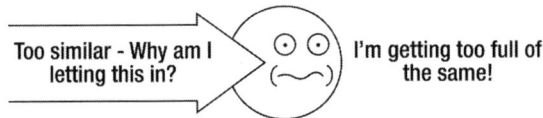

Figure 2.47

Redundancy occurs at every system level: person, member, subgroup and group-as-a-whole systems. It is interesting to note how the energy drops in all systems when they become redundant. When functional subgrouping is working well, one or more members will recognize the shift in energy to redundancy and start to add more differences. Systems-centered therapists can also readily draw the group's attention to the static experience of doing the same thing over and over without any sense of change.

What came before and what comes next

In this chapter, we have explored the life force energy/information that is the fuel for survival, development and transformation. We have also looked at SCT's integration of Shannon and Weaver's (1964) work on noise in the communication channel and its impact on boundary permeability and introduced the arrows as dynamic vectors that carry communications within, between and among the systems in the hierarchy. We reconceptualized vectors as driving and restraining forces building on Lewin (1951) which, when communication vectors are charted in a force field, allows therapists to identify which are the easiest restraining forces to weaken so that the system can move towards its goals. This then gives therapists a game plan to re-vector the system towards its context goals. Re-vectoring applies to all system levels – person, member, subgroup, group-as-a-whole.

Notes

1 The two systems of known and unknown have many roots in the literature. There is the conscious, pre-conscious and unconscious; there are the intellectual, the emotional and the existential; there is the brain–body dimension; and so on into the many allied fields of exploration into human physiology and psychology.
2 In 1965, Anita Simon and I (Yvonne) developed an observation system that was intended to provide an operational definition of Shannon and Weaver's (1964) assumption that there is an inverse relationship between entropic noise in the communication channel and the probability that the information it contained would be transferred. The result was the SAVI Grid (Sequential Analysis of Verbal Interaction) which generated a "map" of the probability that the communication pattern resulting from coding the verbal behaviors would approach or avoid solving the problems inherent in the communication. Reaching the goals of the communication is thus contingent on sufficiently resolving the problems inherent in the communication process.

References

Agazarian, Y. M. (1992). Contemporary theories of group psychotherapy: A systems approach to the group-as-a-whole. *International Journal of Group Psychotherapy*, *42*(3), 177–203. doi:10.1080/00207284.1992.11490685

Agazarian, Y. M. (1997). *Systems-centered therapy for groups*. New York, NY: Guilford Press. Reprinted in paperback (2004). London, UK: Karnac Books.

Lewin, K. (1951). *Field theory in social science*. New York, NY: Harper & Row.

Miller, J. G. (1978). *Living systems*. New York, NY: McGraw-Hill.

Shannon, C. E., & Weaver, W. (1964). *The mathematical theory of communication*. Urbana, IL: University of Illinois Press.

Simon, A., & Agazarian, Y. M. (1967). *SAVI: Sequential analysis of verbal interaction*. Philadelphia, PA: Research for Better Schools.

Simon, A., & Agazarian, Y. M. (2000). SAVI: The system for analyzing verbal interaction. In A. P. Beck & C. M. Lewis (Eds.), *The process of group psychotherapy: Systems for analyzing change* (pp. 357–380). Washington, DC: American Psychological Association.

Chapter 3

Transitions in SCT theory and practice 2013–2016

It is fundamental to SCT that systems-centered therapy is a theory-driven practice. This means that when SCT is put into practice, every intervention tests both the validity of its theory as well as the reliability of its practice. We have found this process both a curse and a blessing. It is a curse because every time we think we have a final version, something happens that seems to contradict the theory, facing us with the challenge to reevaluate our assumptions and review our practice. Thus, the work of developing theory is never done. On the other hand, it is also a blessing because when we become aware of contradictions, we can think again and revise both our theory and our practice. This is a never-ending challenge. Theory is neutral; we are not. Theory constantly challenges us to be objective. We are constantly pulled towards being subjective. Theory requires us to think outside the box, but often we retreat to the comforts of the known, inside the box.

I (Yvonne) have Dave Jenkins, the head of the Group Dynamics Department at Temple University, to thank for this discipline. For two years he tutored me, insisting that I made operational definitions for my theorizing, so that I could test whether or not they were useful in practice. It is thus that I, and many of our SCT practitioners, became informal action researchers as well as theoreticians.

Parenthetically, although I have been the developer of a TLHS, my insights are fundamentally influenced by the work of our SCT theory groups, training groups and therapy groups, and discussions with many SCT practitioners, all of whom are as challenged as I am in the ongoing task of synchronizing theory and practice. SCT is not only a work in progress, but its members also take the roles of field researchers! Thus, I am using "we" as well as "I" throughout the rest of this chapter as we explore some of the new developments in our systems-centered practice.

This chapter introduces our revisions and innovations to our practice of how systems-centered therapy addressed a serious misinterpretation that had crept into our practice. Our misinterpretation arose when we were framing the impact of our personalizing role in systems-centered training and therapy, and the development that happened to both the theory and practice in the process of "trying to put it right"!

Personalizing "personalizing"

I had become personally concerned that, when people took things just personally (in spite of considerable insight into old roles), new roles became unavailable and the old roles took over. Worse than that – I watched our members (and myself) demonstrate that when we took things "just personally" we also seemed to induce others into personalizing as well. This then led to dysfunctional subgrouping.[1] This was our worst nightmare! As functional subgrouping is the major method that translates our theory into systems-centered practice, it was disheartening to observe that in the real world of every day, personalizing led to role locks and "as if" subgrouping rather than to the SCT *functional* subgrouping we depend on as our SCT method for conflict resolution.

Functional subgrouping

The function of functional subgrouping in the practice of SCT is that it is the method that influences the ability to discriminate and integrate *differences* – both a necessary and sufficient dynamic to enable the survival, development and transformation of all living human systems. Therefore, I took it for granted that anything that undermines this dynamic was "always" a restraining force. The more concerned I became, the more I redoubled my efforts to communicate the cost of personalizing to our membership. (However hard I tried, nothing changed!) What is more, I was unaware that in my zeal, I was myself personalizing "personalizing"!

My personal influence attempt!

The following flyer (see Figure 3.1) that I energetically distributed through SCT workshops, groups and the SCTRI newsletter is a good example of the pressure I was inadvertently putting on the membership of SCTRI. It was a good advertisement for "not" personalizing but, like all advertisements, it preached mainly to the converted, and even the converted were finding it difficult to implement!

The wake-up call in our 2013 conference large group

We end every day at our SCT conferences with a large group with all conference participants. As it often happens, the work of the large group emerges not only around issues that are the heart of the conference itself but also around issues important in the development of our organization-as-a-whole: the Systems-Centered Training and Research Institute.

Not taking oneself just personally!

Alert! Taking things just personally is probably the major source of anguish that we experience in our lives! When we take things just personally all we are aware of is ourselves. Everything is all about us! It's like looking at a Russian doll and seeing only oneself in the doll. We are closed systems, with boundariesclosed to exchanges between ourselves and the outside world unless they match what we already believe. Much of our personal anguish comes from personalizing: seeing ourselves as the center of the world.

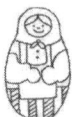

No man is an island. Seeing oneself as a system as well as a person means that we can become aware of the many changing views of the world and can see how we influence the world and the world influences us. We can tell the difference between seeing ourselves from the inside and seeing from the inside out.

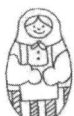

A Russian doll may look like an individual, but in fact it is not. It does not look as if it contains a whole hierarchy of dolls, but in fact it does! To "see" this requires knowing that it does. Both sight and insight!

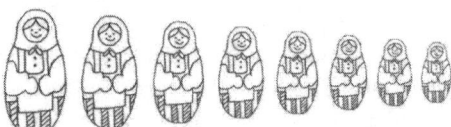

Seeing a Russian doll in a whole hierarchy of nesting dolls changes our world! Once we see the dolls as a series of interconnected systems, several things become obvious. We can see ourselves as part of an isomorphic hierarchy: more similar than different to others who live in the world with us. We can choose any of the doll "systems" to learn more about the doll system that contains our personal core energy, the next doll system that is a member, the doll system that contains the member, the doll system that is a member of a group, a group system that is a member of a larger group, etc., etc., etc., becoming system-centered in a systems-centered world! Seeing ourselves as systems-centered rather than self-centered means that we are aware of the system context that we are in and how it changes as we shift in our world from home to work to play.

Figure 3.1

In 2013, the conflict around personalizing emerged in the large group. Quite spontaneously, the group-as-a-whole began to "train" its members on the difference between "person" and "member" language. In functional subgrouping, we identify a difference between a membership response where one first reflects what the last person just said before building on it, in contrast to personally preempting the communication by responding with a personal response. Reflecting establishes functional subgrouping. Personalized responses establish personalizing.

In this particular large group, when a member in the large group "explained" themselves instead of "exploring" either themselves or their subgroup, the group would identify the personal "explanations and intellectualizations" as a "personalizing" role. This contrasts with feedback from objective, exploratory or attuned communications which contains the necessary curiosity that we all need if we are to become aware of others' contributions as different from our own.

Group working in roles and role lock phase of development

The group's work placed the group-as-a-whole in the roles and role lock phase of system development. (SCT works from a phase model that progresses from flight to fight to roles/role locks to intimacy to work.) The goal in the roles/role lock phase is recognizing and undoing the roles and role locks that happen in the group between members. This work then enables members to test reality by checking whether one's explanations of interpersonal experience are projections from a past or out of context role (that fuels the role lock between the two) or perceptions that reflect reality. By the time the group reaches this phase, the protocol for undoing "mindreading" (in which a member verbalizes their mindread of another member as a yes or no question to test reality) has already been introduced. This protocol is then helpfully used as part of undoing the roles and role locks. It is in the role lock phase that the group members learn to give each other neutral and supportive feedback about the impact of their roles. It is also the phase in which groups learn to identify the role inductions that occur when members personalize, given that personalizing roles are the old roles that were adaptive in the past but rarely in the present. The leaders of the large group were excited by the large group spontaneously working within the role phase, which was a useful step in the development of the group.

Group regression into scapegoating

However, our leadership appreciation of this level of new work was premature. What happened next was a shift in climate. The pressure to shout "person" or "member" increased and the intensity shifted the group from feedback into attack. The group shifted from helpfully training members to acting out fight phase dynamics! This regression from the roles phase to the fight phase subverted the overt intention of "training" group members to the behavior of "scapegoating" group members! Predictably, what replaced supportive sub-grouping were powerful role inductions into dominant and submissive role locks that are inherent to the fight phase. Not surprisingly, working energy was sidelined into surges of sadism and masochism. This was fascinating to us after we got through our shock. Before elaborating, it is useful to quickly review the history of our large groups.

The development of our conference large groups

We have long been interested in large groups (Agazarian & Carter, 1993). It was in the early 1990s in the beginning of systems-centered workshops and conferences when we first convened large groups, and their dynamics were as chaotic as most large groups are in most group conferences. Large groups typically replicate the culture. Culturally, as human beings we tend to man-age the differences between ourselves and others by assuming dominant or submissive role relationships and, like all other animals, we ignore, isolate, attack, scapegoat, and extrude each other for being different from us. Our long history demonstrates that our responses to difference make us the most destructive animals on our planet. (All animals hate differences!) So why in SCT do we say that differences are the source of creative change? Because our theory says all systems survive, develop and transform from simpler to more complex through the discrimination and integration of differences: that is differences in the apparently similar and similarities in the apparently different. In fact, SCT developed functional subgrouping as a conflict reso-lution method to discriminate and integrate differences. Group members are first required to reflect the other's input before introducing one's own response.

When functional subgrouping became the whole system norm in SCT groups, the underlying conflictual dynamics of each developmental phase tended to be contained well enough that the dynamics were sufficiently benign that they could be explored in SCT groups rather than acted out (Agazar-ian, 1994; Agazarian & Gantt, 2003). Especially in our large groups (Gantt & Agazarian, 2011; O'Neill & Mogle, 2015), the benefit was less chaotic group development. The liability was that our participants did not have the learning experiences of the group dynamics that are more typically characteristic of large groups. Thus, using functional subgrouping methods in SCT groups basi-cally contains the underlying dynamics and bypasses the enactments that are so well described by Bion (1961) and Bennis and Shepard (1956). The advantage is that group development is less chaotic. The liability is that SCT groups are less likely to give their members the experience of the acting out that occurs in all groups when the dynamics are uncontained. Thus, SCT groups (with exceptions of course) are not the best arena for learning through experience about the predictable chaos and role inductions that emerge in all phases of most developing groups!

More on our large group enactment

In the conference large group we have been describing, the norms for sub-grouping broke down and chaos reemerged. The group found itself drawn into enacting rather than exploring the flight/fight phases and scapegoating, with the outraged feelings in one subgroup and anxiety and withdrawal in the other. Thus, there were two subgroups and for the first time in many years, the group acted out the fight impulses to scapegoat those who were personalizing instead of containing the impulse and exploring it in subgrouping.

Thus, the group, its members and its leaders had an experience of dysfunctional subgrouping and a live example of what SCT calls a system-as-a-whole dynamic in which members become helpless puppets on the strings of group phase dynamics. This in turn led us to a deeper understanding that roles never exist in a vacuum and are always part of a systemic interaction, either within ourselves, with others or with the context.

Large group review

In the large group review at the end, the group surfaced its concern about creating identified patients and scapegoating them and was awed by how quickly fight dynamics aroused varied impulses within the members, including the impulse to scapegoat. Shocking as the experience was for many of us, the large group review surfaced a range of different responses and insights for both the leaders and its members. Members experienced, firsthand, the impact of two different developmental phases of the group and the difference between them (developing and strengthening reality-testing in the feedback phase and creating identified patients and scapegoats in the phase of flight/fight).

Serendipitously, the group's confrontation of the leaders and the exploration into the various subgroups' reactions paid off. First and foremost, it was the members who introduced the system self-correction that the leaders had missed! Thus, there was evidence that the member–leader boundary was permeable. Second, in the exploratory work that followed, the group linked "prejudice against personalizing" to the scapegoating dynamic that emerged and the "follow-the-leader" dynamic nested in the underlying dependency of the authority phases. This was a useful demonstration of the isomorphic connection between personal bias and system-as-a-whole dynamics. Leadership bias influenced member bias, which influenced both personal bias and the group-as-a-whole. Although at the time we as leaders were still blind, this was to lead us to a highly significant discovery around the system dynamics of personalizing.

Driving and restraining forces: opposing goals

We can say now that we and our members were on the way to recognizing the restraining force of the destructive dynamics that are omnipresent in all groups and that all members of groups, and SCT members in particular, are often under internal pressure to deny these dynamics. Many SCT members had previously acquired intellectual knowledge of the chaos in the dynamics under-lying groups through reading the literature (Freud's *Totem and Taboo* [1918] is an important source of understanding!), but had not yet lived through the chaotic experience of the potential destructiveness in flight/fight, as well as the threats in the phase dynamics in the "crisis of hatred."

The driving forces for us and our members were that the experience opened the door to some essential retraining. Previously, in my own training experiences, gained as both a member and a trainer in Tavistock and A. K. Rice workshops, I developed deep insight into the chaotic undertone in all groups. Tavistock methods, with the deliberately blank face of the leader, are a significant role induction into early responses to the loss of attunement and empathy as Yalom (1995) pointed out. These reactions are established very early and, as Spitz (1965) noted, failures of attunement and resonance in the attachment between infants and care-takers in vulnerable infants is an essential factor in their failure to thrive.

As I had learned in my own experience of "blank face leadership," groups tended to respond in a predictable sequence: first flight-driven anxiety, then targeting and scapegoating, followed by interpersonal conflict and finally culminating in the crisis of hatred in which the group-as-a-whole directs paranoid projections at the leader (Agazarian, 1997; Bennis & Shepard, 1956). In my own experiences of learning how to stay open to my underlying annihilation anxiety in this phase, I did indeed experience what Freud so aptly describes in his *Totem and Taboo* (1918) as the visceral threat of being "killed and eaten!" I know that this is also true for many of us who contain the group dynamics in the group crisis of hatred.

Remembering that driving and restraining forces are goal-directed

Luckily, there was also a positive outcome in how we came to understand the unexpected dynamics in this large group. Out of the chaos came a recall of neglected theory! We remembered Lewin's (1951) emphasis that all driving and restraining forces are goal-directed. Driving forces orient the system to the goals of development; restraining forces orient the system to the goals of maintaining stability. Both are necessary in the system development process. Thus, the restraining force of "personalizing" was also a driving force towards an opposite goal. Our challenge was to define and legitimize the goal of per-sonalizing as equally important.

Conference consequences: new theory – new illustrations – new practice

For me personally, remembering the importance of driving and restraining forces in maintaining group stability on the one hand and moving the system towards or away from developmental goals on the other began a two-year experience of living in the chaos of the unknown. I apprehensively knew that we were confronted with an important change in apprehensive understanding – without any connection to the words that would explain it. The illustrations that had clarified my thinking before no longer seemed to be illustrating what I was trying to intuit. In the following two years of theoretical chaos, our theory groups and I drew and redrew illustrations of what we were trying to find words for. We were in a wordless, apprehensive experience "at the edge of the unknown." This has its own challenges. On the one hand, there is the excitement of being at the edge of new knowledge and understanding. On the other hand, there is the experience of being at the edge of chaos and the fear of annihilation. And there is even a subgroup of wanting to explain away the need for change. As a matter of interest to some of us, we now reproduce the original three illustrations that represent our person, member and group (see Figure 3.2).

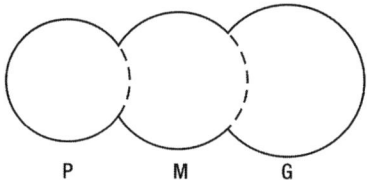

Figure 3.2

Between 2014 and 2016, new ways of thinking came and went as we explored how to illustrate our new ideas about a TLHS and its systems-centered practice. As we drew and redrew, we found our illustrations wanting something more – or less or different – or discovered important connections missing. We kept changing, revising and starting all over again as we worked to elaborate theory that would support undoing "personalizing" the person system. Our eventual solution is obvious now, though not then, and that is to use systems theory to elaborate the system of the person. This solution led us to define our person system as three systems together in one integrated system that we called our whole person (see Figure 3.3).

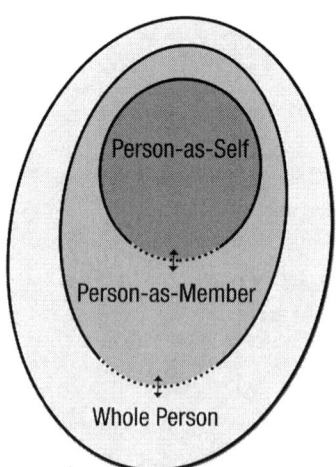

Figure 3.3

First new illustration 2014: personalizing systems!

In the first new illustration that finally emerged, we addressed our "personalizing" dilemma by humanizing our descriptors to make them more personal! We introduced the terms "person-as-self," "person-as-member" and "whole person." This change was well received by trainees and members and SCT patients and accepted as much more user-friendly. There was even a particularly gratifying endorsement from one member who asked "did you change the illustration just for me, or was it that you changed the illustration because you changed your theory?"

This new illustration also made it easier to see the triadic nature of all systems in the hierarchy and easier to recognize that although the function of each system and the goals of each of the three systems are different, the way each system is structured and the dynamics of each system's function are equivalent.

Similarities in the apparently different

In spite of the obvious differences between our pre- and post-2014 illustrations, they have much in common. In both, each of the three systems is unique and also interdependent. All systems are fueled by energy and each different system organizes energy differently. Each system has a goal vectored towards system development, and each plays an important role in system-as-a-whole development. The dynamics that enable each system to vector their energy towards their goals are the same. The permeability of their boundaries is influenced by the same variables. And, most important, because of system isomorphy, what works in one system in any one context will also work for all systems in all contexts! Conceptually, looking at systems from the perspective of isomorphy is like looking into a reflecting mirror: however into the far distance the images go, they never disappear! Drawing all three systems into one containing system seemed to us to make it easier to visualize that (see Figure 3.4).

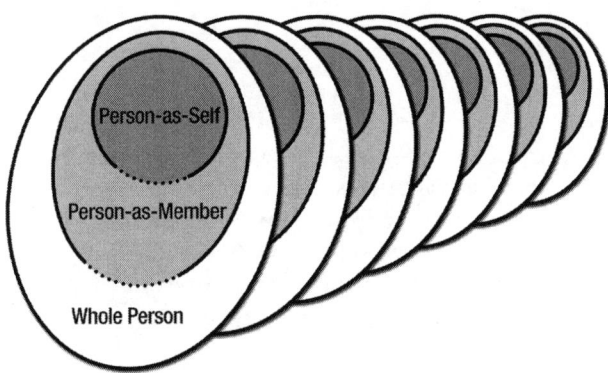

Figure 3.4

Differences in the apparently similar

There are, however, some crucial differences from our original drawings. Our most important change in the way we illustrated our person-as-a-system was using a single circle as the container for the three separate circles that we had used before. A major benefit of introducing our drawings as three nesting circles is that it makes it easier to illustrate our person system as a triad (see Figure 3.3).

We could then see the whole person as the source of all system hierarchies (see Figure 3.5).

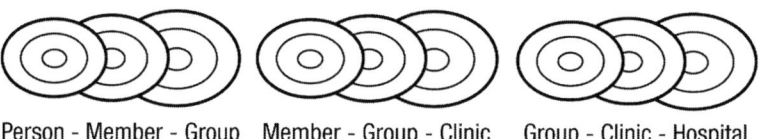

Person - Member - Group   Member - Group - Clinic   Group - Clinic - Hospital

Figure 3.5

Thus, it is not only "not useful" but also essential to refrain from thinking about any one system as if it is alone and to keep in mind that there is always a relationship between it and the system below it and the system above it, returning to our analogy of Russian nesting dolls.

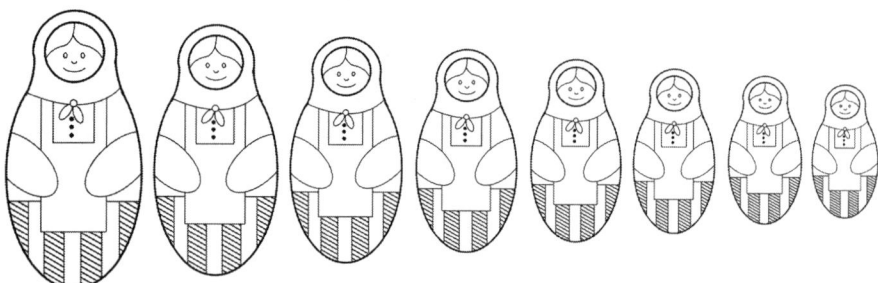

Figure 3.6

The simplicity of this first new drawing was its major contribution. Theoretically, it not only makes it easier to see the triadic nature of all systems in the hierarchy; it also makes it easier to recognize that although the goals of each of the three systems in our new illustration (see Figure 3.3) are different, the way each system is structured and the dynamics of each system's function are equivalent from our individual person-as-a-system and in every system in the hierarchy.

Our first new illustration: our person-as-a-system

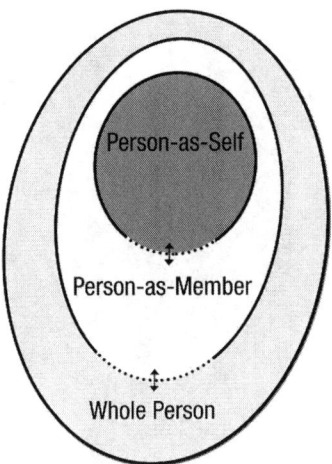

Figure 3.7

Our original "new" illustration had changed the titles of our three systems to make them more user-friendly. (Unfortunately, it was at the expense of linking them explicitly to systems – a reflection of the theoretical confusion I was in after our wake-up call!)

Our person-as-self

"Person-as-self" (see Figure 3.7) was a popular change among most of us who had been uncomfortable about how roles arising from personal experience had been marginalized and scapegoated. There was a new sense of our person being essential to developing a sense of self that deepens through personal experience. With the new descriptor, we legitimized thinking about our person in ways that "feel" like "me" and also the ways that don't feel like me, so that we could also become aware of "that is not me!" We felt that we had introduced a sense of our essential person-as-self, identifying it as essential in the sense that it is the "essence" for developing a sense of self that deepens through personal emotional experience. Personal experience comes first and words come second. It is also true that personalizing makes everything all about me and that reality was later to move us towards a second illustration.

Person-as-member

We defined a new and crucial difference between our person-as-self and our person-as-member (see Figure 3.8).

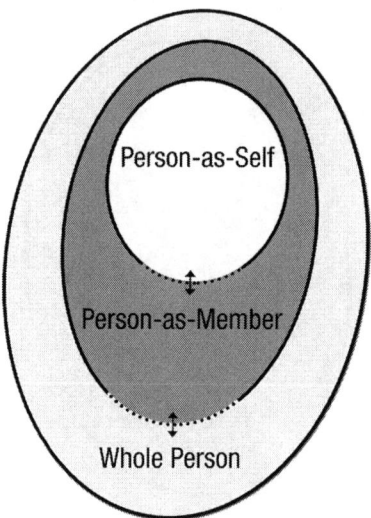

Figure 3.8

When we are living in our person–as–self system, we relate to the context of *our* experience. In our person–as–member, we cross the boundary between ourselves and our member selves. The best example is when we subgroup functionally, in which our first step to person–as–member is to reflect what "the other" has said (this is our inter–person self!) before we join with what is stimulated in us in our person–as–self system and then when we give it to the group by saying it into the group. This helped us to recognize the difference between personal contexts and member contexts, which in turn led us to become more aware of the differences in how our roles change as the system context changes and made it easier to experience the influence of the context shifts on our roles: like the differences in our roles when we are in the context of work, the context of home, and the context of play.

Whole person

When we look at our outer whole person system (see Figure 3.9), we can see that it is the containing system of our triad.

It organizes the energy/information inputs from the middle system and develops the norms that characterize the structure of the person system–as–a–whole. Its goal is to transform from simpler to more complex. Its functional role is norm-setter for the hierarchy and member of the next system triad and so on, up the hierarchy, all fueled by the person system energy.

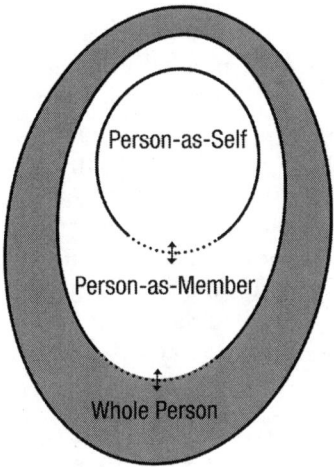

Figure 3.9

Person system and group system

This enabled us to see how the person system energy is the energy system for the hierarchy of not only the person system but also the group system and in turn all isomorphic systems (see Figure 3.10).

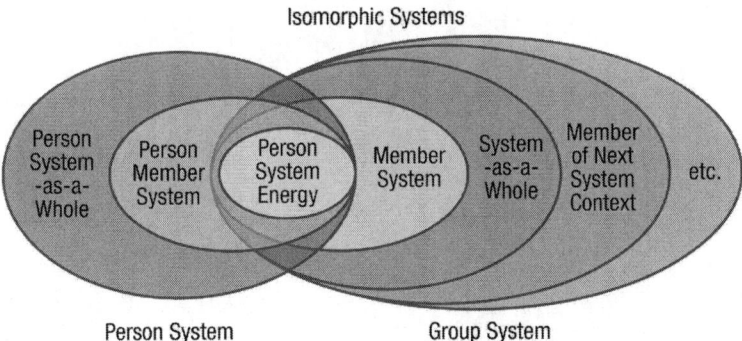

Figure 3.10

Advantages and disadvantages of our first new illustration

By reorganizing our thinking in our new illustration (Figure 3.3), we had managed to legitimately "personalize" our experience so that we could "personally" recognize it, but this came at a cost. As personally satisfying as our new illustration was, we were confronted as theoreticians by the reality that we had personalized our illustration at the expense of a systems theory orientation. We had not only personalized our illustration, we had also oversimplified it.

This was a painful recognition. We asked ourselves whether, in the service of legitimizing personalizing, the modification had been at the expense of recognizing the importance of the system dynamics that are the nexus of systems-centered theory and practice. Our original orientation to systems thinking was in the service of humanizing, legitimizing, normalizing and particularly de-pathologizing our common human dynamics. We would not reach that goal unless we translated our human dynamics into systems language and back again: by defining the necessary de-pathologizing, operational definitions for SCT practice. We therefore reluctantly modified the personalizing comfort of our first set of labels that connected the system directly to ourselves and introduced labels that better reflected a systems perspective.

Our second new illustration: introducing inner-person and inter-person as systems

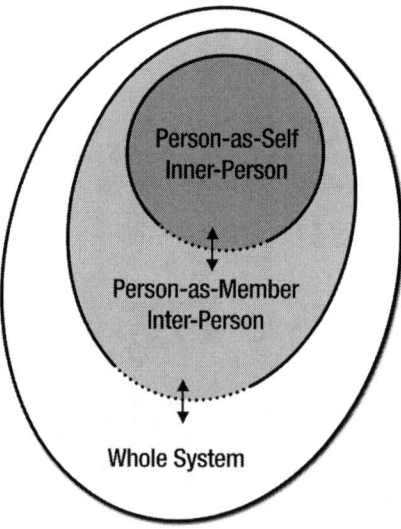

Figure 3.11

First, we substituted "system" descriptors for our personal ones: inner-person for person-as-self, inter-person for person-as-member, and whole system for whole person (see Figure 3.11). This change was a necessary step in depersonalizing our first drawing by restoring a systems orientation in our second drawing! The change allowed us to contrast our inner, curious, self-aware self that related to the energy of our inner self with the energy that relates interpersonally with others. Inter-personal systems are dependent on the context, and membership is related to the goals of the context. Thus, whereas the goal of the inner-person system is system survival, the goal of the inter-person system is system development. We did not know it then, but we were at the beginning of another revolution in our recognition that we had left out some important aspects of our understanding of our new drawings.

Our third new illustration: how we marginalized energy and put it back again

In our third illustration (see Figure 3.12), we labeled the illustration as our person-as-a-system and added energy into our illustration. Yet in another moment of unwelcome insight, we were startled to recognize that we had identified the energy that fueled the person-as-self system in the margin of the drawing and had failed to define how the two energies related to the person systems inside the drawing!

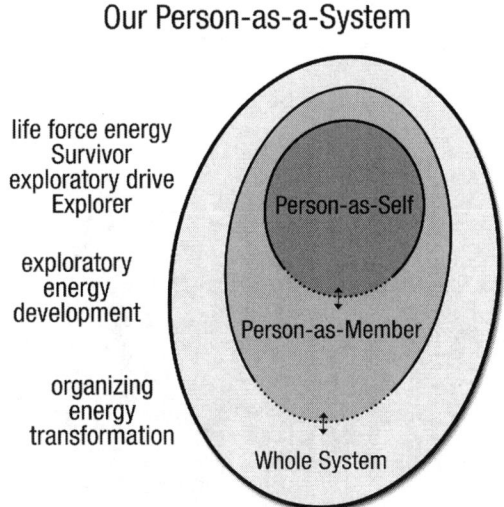

Figure 3.12

By locating both the life force and the exploratory drive in the margin outside the system, we had not had to ask ourselves how these two essential energies actually related to the survival, development and transformation of our inner-person, our inter-person and our whole person (see Figure 3.13).

Changing the drawing helped! Adding a line that linked the energy and the goal to each system (see Figure 3.14) helped us to really "see" the energy that was fundamental to each system of our person-as-a-system.

Our Person-as-a-System

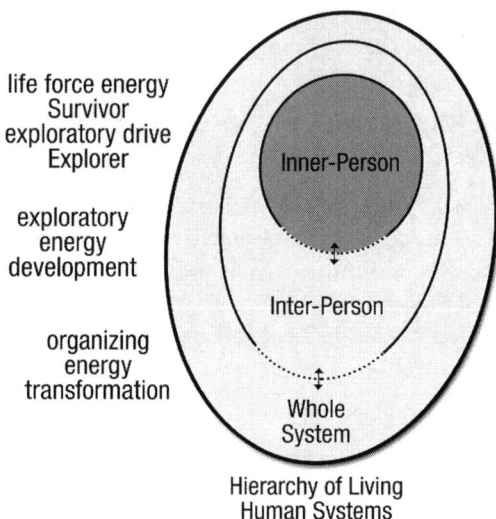

life force energy
Survivor
exploratory drive
Explorer

exploratory
energy
development

organizing
energy
transformation

Inner-Person

Inter-Person

Whole
System

Hierarchy of Living
Human Systems

Figure 3.13

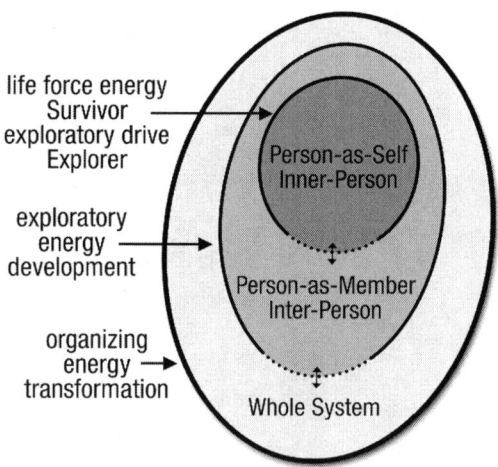

life force energy
Survivor
exploratory drive
Explorer

exploratory
energy
development

organizing
energy
transformation

Person-as-Self
Inner-Person

Person-as-Member
Inter-Person

Whole System

Figure 3.14

Incorporating this line to connect the life force and the exploratory drive to the systems *inside* the drawing led to our next step. We were then able to recognize that we would need to define the dynamic interaction of the life force and the exploratory drive and its impact on system development if we were to understand the development of the inner-person system. This in turn led us to explore the dynamics involved if our inner-person system was to survive, let alone develop and transform. We would also need to consider that, though the life force and the exploratory drive are interdependent energies for system development, each would have important differences for us to take into account in defining the survival of living human systems.

The life force and the exploratory drive: interdependent and different energies

Both the life force and the exploratory drive are energies in the inner-person system with its goal of survival. Whereas the life force depends upon the exploratory drive if the life force is to fuel system development, the exploratory drive depends upon the energy of the life force if it is to actively explore! These two energies are interdependent. We need both life force energy and curiosity if we are to survive and develop as both systems and as people. This opened the door to more innovations!

Our first challenge was to further develop our understanding of the new system that contained the life force and our second was to define the new subsystem that contained the exploratory drive (see Figure 3.15). Survival depends upon the energy of the life force and is necessary for the survival of all systems in our hierarchy of living human systems. Development depends upon the energy of the exploratory drive, necessary for the development and transformation of each system in the hierarchy. Thus, we have introduced two subsystems to make a "home" for the two essential but different energies, each of which have similar, but not the same, drive to their goals!

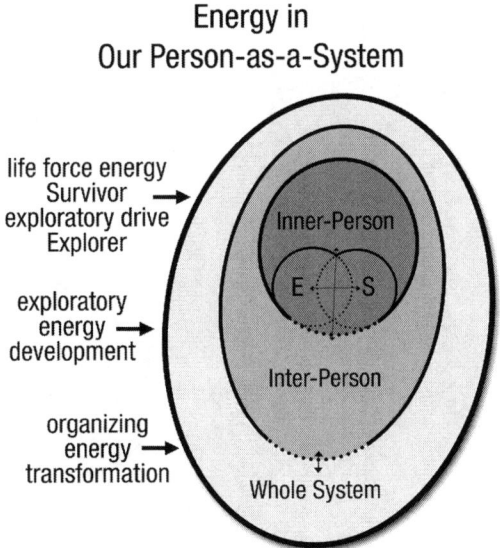

**Energy in
Our Person-as-a-System**

life force energy
Survivor ➞
exploratory drive
Explorer

exploratory
energy ➞
development

organizing
energy ➞
transformation

Inner-Person

E ⬦ S

Inter-Person

Whole System

Figure 3.15

Introducing subsystems of the life force "survivor" and the exploratory drive "explorer"

We allocated the primary energy of the life force to the survivor system. We named it the "survivor," in that the life force is essential for the survival of all living human systems. We allocated the developmental energy of the exploratory drive to the system of the curious explorer. We named it "curious explorer," as it requires curiosity to motivate us to explore the different contexts that influence our ability to survive. These two subsystems are similar in that they both contain energies that are essential to the survival, development and transformation of the inner-person system. They are different in that, though the survivor system can survive (in the short run) without the exploratory drive, the inner-person system can neither develop nor mature without interactions between both.

The survivor system contains the primary energy of the life force and the curious explorer system contains the developmental energy of the exploratory drive. Our next step was to define these two new subsystems, each of which is different, each of which has different energy, each of which has different goals, and both of which are essential to our survival, development and transformation. We need *both* to fuel system survival, development and transformation!

It was in rethinking the inner-person system dynamics that it became clear that experiencing our inner-person without words is different from becoming curious about how our inner-person role-systems developed. We need both subjective person-centered apprehension and subjective curiosity as well as more objective curiosity. Thus, we have our two systems: our central person system contains both the survivor system, which is necessarily subjective, and the curious explorer system, which is subjective and organizes the energy that fuels objectivity in our inter-person systems.

We illustrated this (see Figure 3.16) to show how each role-system with its different goals also contains a different energy. The important implication is that the exploratory drive is as essential to our personal survival as the life force itself.

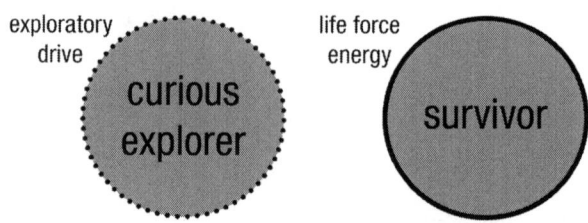

Figure 3.16

Exploring our two inner-person subsystems

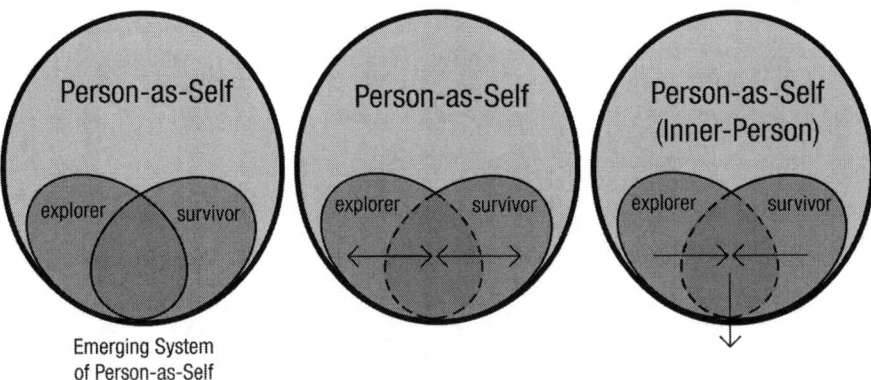

Figure 3.17

A still new illustration (see Figure 3.17) helped us deepen our understanding of the interdependence of the inner-person subsystems of explorer and survivor. Most important was the recognition that development of the survivor system depends upon the explorer to test reality, not just survive "reality"! Only with permeable boundaries, as in the middle illustration, is there potential for the development of a new system in the inner-person system!

Closed and open survivor systems

System survival depends upon recognizing and integrating tolerable differences. Thus, the goal of the survivor system is to prevent intolerable differences from destabilizing it. As we have said, integrating new information is necessary if systems are to develop, but system survival is at stake when differences are so different that they threaten to disrupt the internal equilibrium of the system. When all goes well, the survivor system becomes an open system, which can titrate boundaries to open or close dependent on the context. When all does not go well, it closes its boundaries and becomes a closed system. The inner-person open system is called the open survivor system, a driving force to development. The inner-person closed system is called the closed survivor system, a driving force for survival but a restraining force to development.

Closed survivor system boundaries are closed to our curiosity and therefore also to our exploratory energy. When we are not curious, we remain behind closed boundaries and when our survivor system boundaries are closed, nothing can change! Thus, although closed survivor system boundaries allow our system to survive in the short run, without the exploratory ability to discriminate and integrate differences, we can survive but we cannot thrive. Thus, when our survivor system is closed, we can only survive, but can neither develop nor transform as our boundary is closed to difference. In contrast, our open survivor role-systems are open to the exploratory drive and can develop and transform so that the life force energy in our survivor roles can be more available to our inner-person development and in our inter-person contexts (see Figure 3.18).

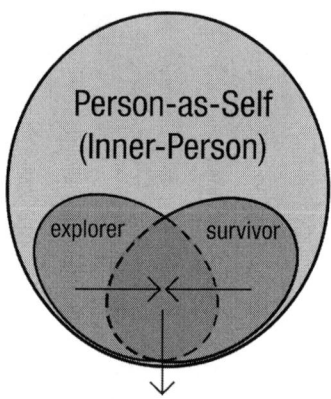

Figure 3.18

The roles that we develop in our survivor self when responding to an experienced threat now have a name. They are called survivor roles, developed at the boundary between the inner-person system and significant others. Survivor role-systems develop to contain the conflict between the threats of differences that arise from failures of resonant affiliation. This occurs, of course, when the personal self preempts the affiliation self. It also occurs when the child is confronted by the socializing demands of their significant others, empathy fails and resonance and attunement become contingent on compliance. Both of these are experienced as a threat!

The importance of curiosity

It is through our exploratory curiosity and our explorer fueling our researcher roles in our inter-person system that we can gather objective information to add to our all-important and essential subjective experience. The particularly important feature of the curious explorer system is that it has the capacity to develop roles that can cross the boundaries and influence the development of the survivor system and can also itself develop more complex roles that can cross the boundaries into the inter-person system.

This in turn implies that curiosity is a necessary (but not sufficient!) role-system signal for change. Thus, the system challenge is to develop an SCT blueprint that guides us to influence a working relationship between our survivor and our curious explorer so that our inner-person system can develop. Integrating these understandings of the inner-person system led us to the next version of our illustration. When this illustration emerged, we found ourselves following an intuitive quantum jump in both our theory and practice!

Our fourth illustration

In this fourth version of our person-as-a-system (see Figure 3.19), we have shifted from our earlier simpler versions to one that helps us explore three additional questions.

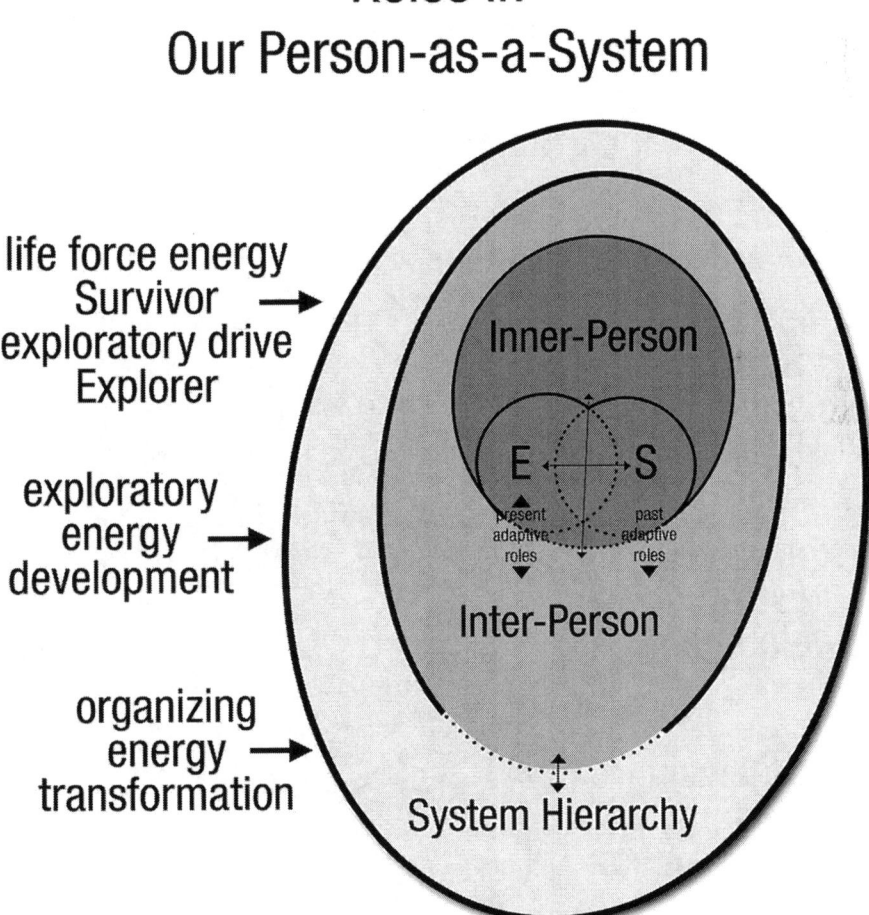

Figure 3.19

The first question is: what does it mean that we have defined the inner-person system as containing two different subsystems called the personal survivor system and the curious explorer system whose outputs are present and past adaptive role-systems?

The second question is: what does it mean for SCT practice that we have introduced the idea that we can think about roles as systems?

The third question is: what does it mean for SCT practice that we are reframing roles not only as systems but also as system outputs which, we will argue, allows us to intuit the goals of their source system?

In our next three chapters, we explore these questions with our newest work (see Figure 3.20) on this blueprint. Chapter 4 picks up the further theoretical exploration that the illustration precipitated us to take, while Chapters 5 and 6 introduce the subsequent innovations in our practice of SCT.

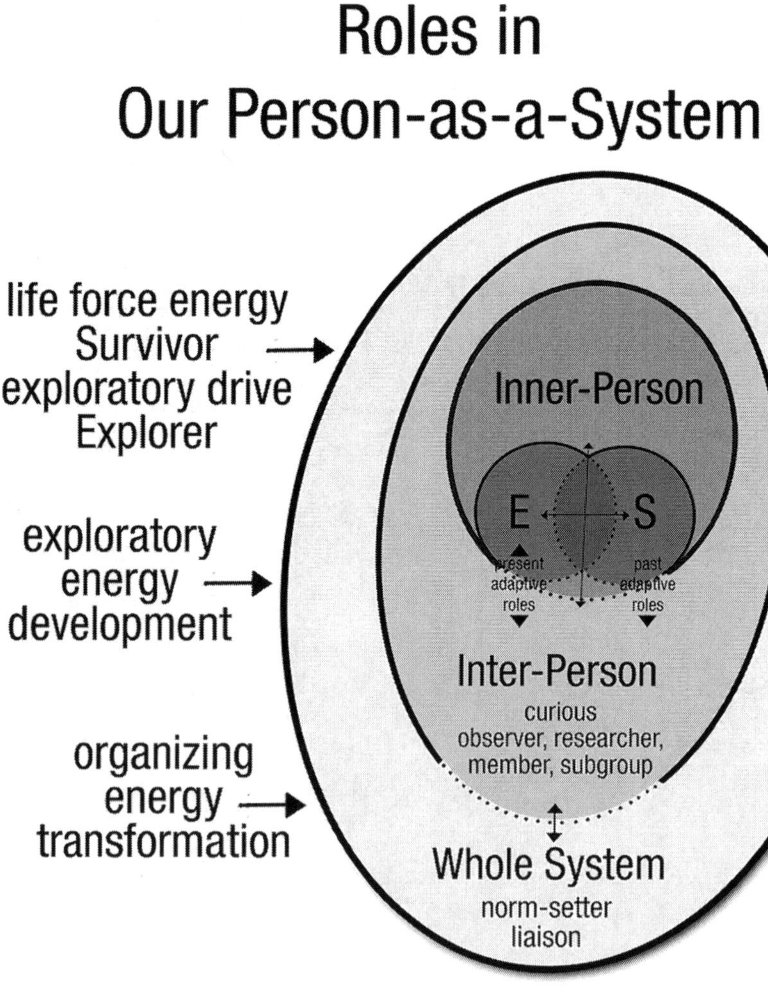

Roles in
Our Person-as-a-System

Figure 3.20

Note

1 Dysfunctional can be traumatic: when the words don't "match the music," when the face is blank, when the words are "right" but the emotion is not. This is a graphic example of how not only do "words without feeling" have no meaning but also "words without feeling" arouse distrust and can invite a paranoid role response.

References

Agazarian, Y. M. (1994). The phases of development and the systems-centered group. In M. Pines & V. Schermer (Eds.), *Ring of fire: Primitive object relations and affect in group psychotherapy* (pp. 36–85). London, UK: Routledge, Chapman & Hall.

Agazarian, Y. M. (1997). *Systems-centered therapy for groups*. New York, NY: Guilford Press. Reprinted in paperback (2004). London, UK: Karnac Books.

Agazarian, Y. M., & Carter, F. (1993). The large group and systems-centered theory. *GROUP: The Journal of the Eastern Group Psychotherapy Society, 17*(4), 210–234.

Agazarian, Y. M., & Gantt, S. P. (2003). Phases of group development: Systems-centered hypotheses and their implications for research and practice. *Group Dynamics: Theory, Research and Practice, 7*(3), 238–252. doi:10.1037/1089-2699.7.3.238

Bennis, W. G., & Shepard, H. A. (1956). A theory of group development. *Human Relations, 9*(4), 415–437. doi:10.1177/001872675600900403

Bion, W. R. (1961). *Experiences in groups*. London, UK: Tavistock.

Freud, S. (1918). *Totem and taboo* (A. A. Brill, Trans.). New York, NY: Moffat, Yard.

Gantt, S. P., & Agazarian, Y. M. (2011). Highlights from ten years of a systems-centered large group: Work in progress. *Voices: The Art and Science of Psychotherapy, 47*(1), 40–50.

Lewin, K. (1951). *Field theory in social science*. New York, NY: Harper & Row.

O'Neill, R. M., & Mogle, J. (2015). Systems-centered functional subgrouping and large group outcome. *GROUP: The Journal of the Eastern Group Psychotherapy Society, 39*(4), 303–317. doi:10.13186/group.39.4.0303

Spitz, R. A. (1965). *The first year of life: A psychoanalytic study of normal and deviant development of object relations*. New York, NY: International Universities Press.

Yalom, I. D. (1995). *The theory and practice of group psychotherapy* (4th ed.). New York, NY: Basic Books.

Role-systems: Theory and implications

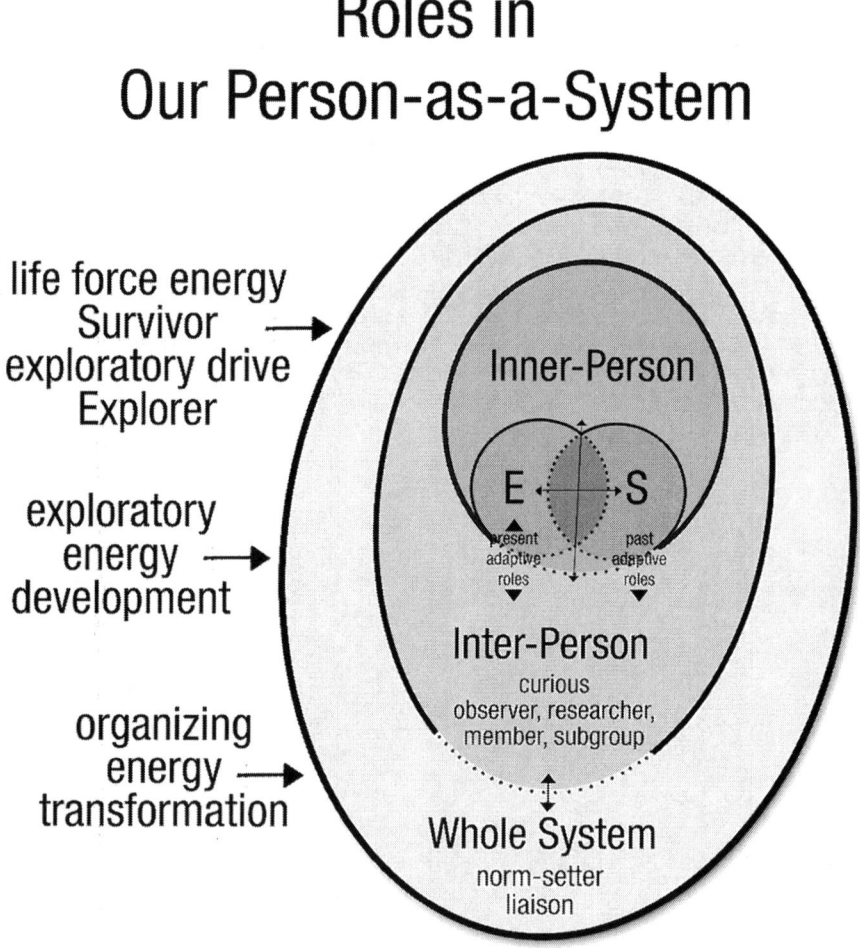

Figure 4.1

We have for some time referred to roles as systems, yet prior to the work described in Chapter 3, we had not really developed our understanding of roles themselves as systems and the implications of defining roles as living human systems. This is our major innovation in this chapter: defining roles as living human systems, which means that every role can be defined in terms of a hierarchy of isomorphic systems that are energy-organizing, goal-directing and self-correcting (see Figure 4.1). This work is now revolutionizing how we think about systems-centered practice.

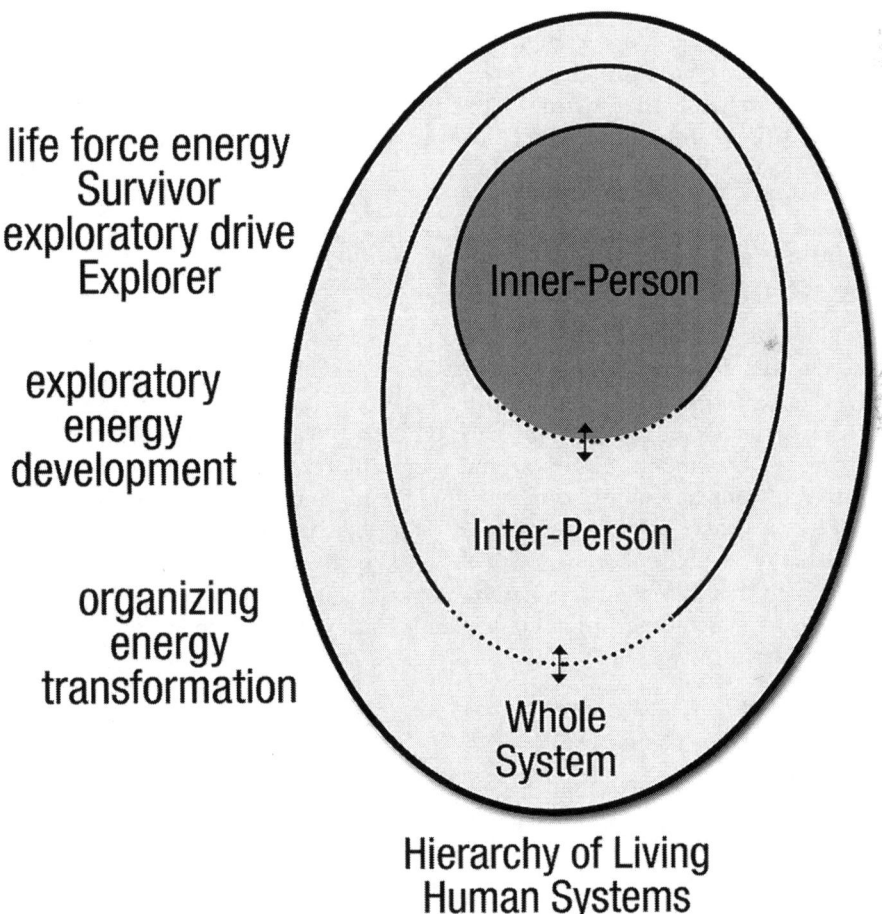

Our Person-as-a-System

life force energy
Survivor
exploratory drive
Explorer

exploratory
energy
development

organizing
energy
transformation

Inner-Person

Inter-Person

Whole
System

Hierarchy of Living
Human Systems

Figure 4.2

Defining roles as living human systems that exist in an isomorphic hierarchy

It is a major bonus for us that by redefining roles as systems, we can then assume that roles and role dynamics in this defined hierarchy are isomorphic: similar in structure (how they manage the permeability of their boundaries) and in function (how they discriminate and integrate differences). Thus, by defining role-systems as isomorphic we can identify the common dynamics that generalize to all role-systems, whatever their derivation. Looking at the illustration (see Figure 4.2) helps us see how each system in our triad of systems shares the same structure and functions in the same way as every other system in the hierarchy and yet, paradoxically, each is also unique! In addition, because roles are systems, and systems are isomorphic, methods that work in influencing the structure or function of any one role-system will work with every other role-system at every level of the hierarchy – person, member, small and larger groups, and so on up the hierarchy of living human systems. In recognizing common dynamics, we can also generalize to predicted outcomes from the roles that people play in other contexts, or the roles that groups, organizations and nations play in their contexts.

Roles as "goal-directing, energy-organizing and self-correcting" systems

As a hierarchy of isomorphic systems, our person-as-a-system is goal-directing, energy-organizing and self-correcting. Our illustration (see Figure 4.2) is also useful here in that it makes it relatively easy to recognize that different systems in this hierarchy of role-systems have different goals and roles. We had long recognized that member role outputs were different than person system outputs. With our new illustration, we could easily intuit that output from roles that contain survival system goals will be visibly different from the output of roles that relate to developmental goals of the inter-person system and different again from the roles related to system-as-a-whole transformations. This was an exciting understanding for us, which leads us to exploring the implications of seeing roles as goal-directing systems.

Role-systems are goal-directing

Like all living human systems, role-systems have a goal! This was important in helping us rethink when we recognized that we had diagnosed "personalizing" as a restraining force. This rethinking led us to remember that in a force field, every restraining force is also balanced by a driving force, and vice versa. Once again, we were guided by applying Lewin's (1951) theory that whether or not a goal-directing force is driving or restraining depends not upon the force itself, but the goals. As we know, Lewin states that all forces in his force field drive towards a goal: driving forces drive towards one particular goal and the opposing, restraining forces drive towards an equal and opposite goal. Thus, it follows that whether a role is a driving or a restraining force depends not upon the roles themselves, but upon whether the role is driving or restraining in relation to the goals of its context. A driving force towards one goal will be a restraining force towards another and vice versa!

Whether or not "personalizing" (which, at the theory level, is closing boundaries to any context except our "person") can function as a driving or restraining force depends upon the goals *of its context*. The challenge then was, after we recognized our overemphasis on the personalizing role as a restraining force (see Chapter 3), how could we conceptualize the goals for which a personalizing role-system is a driving force? This took us to identifying the implicit goal of personalizing, which is to stabilize and keep out differences that destabilize. This recognition made it easy to understand and appreciate the function of closing boundaries for stability.

Using the force field model allows us to assume that increasing a driving force or weakening a restraining force will change not only the system's equilibrium but also the system's relationship to its goals. Lewin (1951) stressed that weakening restraining forces leads to change that is more sustainable as the system makes a new equilibrium each time a restraining force is weakened. Lewin also recognized and demonstrated that it is easier to influence the potential for moving towards or away from a goal by weakening the restraining forces than by increasing the driving forces. This has long been standard practice in SCT. For example, SCT anxiety protocols reduce the negative predictions about the future before exploring what it is in the present that is fearful: SCT calls this reducing the paper tigers so that we can see whether a real tiger is there! Attempting to reality-test (a driving force) whether there are real tigers before undoing the negative predictions about paper tigers (restraining forces to reality-testing) is quite difficult! This has been important to us in SCT practice where we work with a hierarchy of defense modification where we weaken restraining forces that are phase-relevant to free the resources that are essential for developing in the specific phase context. This is particularly important in our new work with roles as systems, which we elaborate in Chapter 5 and link to the context of phases of system development in Chapter 9.

In the force field here (see Figure 4.3), we have identified driving and restraining forces in personalizing roles (again, in theory language, these are roles with relatively closed boundaries) where the goal is stability. As with all force fields, this one depicts a system in "quasi-stationary equilibrium" with equal and opposite forces.

Force Field	
DRIVING FORCES IN → PERSONALIZING ROLES	← RESTRAINING FORCES IN PERSONALIZING ROLES
Closing boundaries to differences to → reduce the destabilizing threats to system survival	← Maintaining boundaries impermeable to the transfer of new information
Closing boundaries to all explorer and → curious observer roles including those roles that contain just noticeable differences within compatible similarity	← Closing boundaries at the expense of development

Figure 4.3

Whether a role-system is a driving or a restraining force depends not upon the roles themselves, but upon the goal. In this force field where the goal is survival, closing boundaries to differences is an important driving force. In contrast, if the goal is development, all the driving forces listed in this force field would in fact be restraining forces, as closing boundaries to differences restrains development because development requires discriminating and integrating differences.

This expanded our understanding of how different role-systems had different goals with then different driving and restraining forces. Thus, the force field for survival system goals in the inner-person will be visibly different from the force field that relates to developmental goals of the inter-person system and different again from the force field related to system-as-a-whole transformations. This then led us to further exploration of how driving and restraining forces are reflected in role-system outputs. Our insight as we continued to consider this also led us to excogitate again about vectors as we recognized that a vector's "point of application" is different from a system's goal! This required us to rethink our use of vectors in relationship to role-system goals.

Rethinking vectors

Prior to developing our theory of role-systems, we had used the idea of vectors to describe how energy/information was transferred between and among systems, as we discussed in Chapter 2. Defining the arrows that convey energy/information between systems as vectors had been useful to us in linking theory and practice. We had assigned vectors the role of transferring energy from one system to another across boundaries within, between and among our system triads within the hierarchy. We had defined vectors as having a direction, energy, velocity and a point of application (we assumed the point of application could be redefined as a goal). However, our original understanding of vectors did not take into account the origin of the energy/information that the vector contained. Nor did it consider whether the energy/information the vectors contained would be received at their point of application; that is, we had not looked at the connection to either the sending or receiving systems.

In this process of discovering role-systems, we arrived at a different insight that permanently changed the way we thought about vectors. We replaced our original definition of vectors with the definitions for isomorphic role-systems. This added a new variable to our understanding of how energy/information is transferred within and across the boundaries of all systems. By integrating Lewin's (1951) insight that the output of a system contains the same goals as the system from which it originates, each role-system is an output that links to its originating system. What is more, because role-systems are outputs, we could assume that they had the same goals as their system of origin.

Our new solution is the idea that the transfer of energy/information can be better understood if it is viewed as a role-system that contains the organizations of energy/information that are vectored. From our new perspective, the arrows that cross the boundaries between systems now are represented as role-systems (see Figure 4.4).

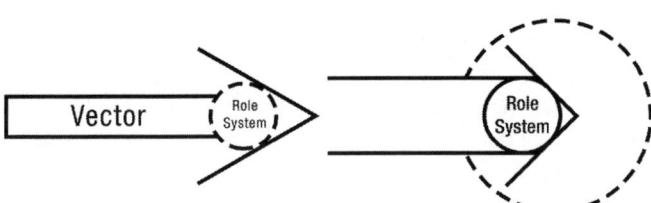

Figure 4.4

We have redefined the meaning of the word "vector" to represent role-systems that cross the boundaries between systems and transfer energy/information from the "sending system" to the "receiving system" (see Figure 4.5). This developed a new dimension to our systems thinking and understanding of role-systems.

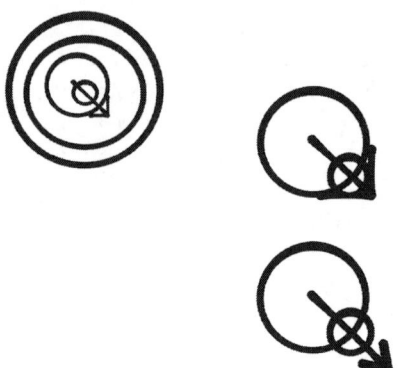

Figure 4.5

This new understanding had roots in our earlier work. For example, we have long been interested in communications as identifying role patterns. Since the early 1990s, we have used our SAVI system for analyzing verbal interactions to identify system communication patterns from the different ways that people talk (their "verbal" behavior!) (Simon & Agazarian, 1967). At the 1992 American Group Psychotherapy Association conference, Yvonne analyzed two of Yalom's tapes illustrating his approach to group work to introduce the connection between the role induction of a leadership style and the induction of group members into functional or nonfunctional subgroups (Agazarian, 1992). In this analysis, she used the SAVI analysis to code the communication patterns. The first of Yalom's tapes were coded as patterns consistent with inducing the role of the "identified patient" and the second inducing the role of "scapegoat"! Even earlier, in Yvonne's 1981 book (Agazarian & Peters, 1981) with Dick Peters, she had worked with the input/output relationships among person, member, role and group. Our new understanding both fit well and extended our earlier work, as this was all before we had role-system theory to guide us!

Role-systems as outputs of their source system

Applying Lewin's (1951) ideas to role-systems, we can then say that when we define roles as system outputs, we can intuit the goal of the originating system by observing the characteristics of the role behavior. Role-systems then not only convey the energy/information across boundaries between systems but also contain the *goals* of the sending or originating system. Thus, from observing role *behavior* in our human world from a systems-centered perspective, we can intuit the *goals* of our roles by recognizing their characteristic behaviors. We can then locate our roles in the relevant system context: inner-person, inter-person or whole system. We can also identify for which system goals a role itself is a driving or restraining force. For example, if the role is a personalizing role, we can judge that it is a driving force in closing inner-person survival system boundaries to a destabilizing threat, but we can also see it as a restraining force to inner-person survivor system development.

For example, the curious explorer role can be identified by a person's curious behavior, necessary for insight, when working with survivor roles in the inner-person system! Recognizing whether a patient is curious will determine whether he or she is closed or open to change. Similarly, with a work group, curiosity often signals readiness for innovative ideas or lack thereof, which signals retrenchment goals.

Reflection of the other's message before contributing one's own is characteristic of inter-person role behavior with a functional subgrouping role. The goal of inner-person roles is to develop the self, whereas the goal of inter-person roles is to develop the context as a containing and developing system (role, goal, context!).

Sending and receiving systems and their boundaries

These understandings also enabled us to connect the goals of the sending system which develops the role to how permeable the boundaries of the receiving system are to the energy/information the role-system conveys. Thus, role-systems developed in the inner-person system which relate to inner-person goals will impact receiving boundaries differently from those developed in the inter-person system with inter-person goals and different again from system-as-a-whole goals. Similarly, closed survivor roles will impact receiving boundaries differently than the open survivor role outputs (see Figure 4.6).

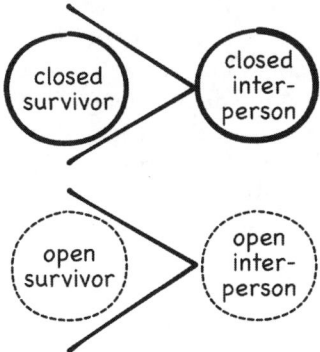

Figure 4.6

Furthermore, using Lewin's (1951) formulation allows us to think not only about the originating system but also about how the implicit goals of the sending system relate to whether the boundaries of the receiving system are permeable to their energy/information. We could assume if the receiving system closed its boundaries to a role-system output from the sending system that this output contained a threat to the receiving system's equilibrium. Or, put simply, receiving systems close boundaries to output that is too different to receive! Thus, closing boundaries to threat is a driving force for system survival and a restraining force to system development, and both survival and development are essential to the survival, development and transformation of all living human systems. All systems center around homeostasis! As we have stressed in SCT, we use Lewin's construct of the force field to illustrate homeostasis as a function of an equilibrium between opposite and equal driving and restraining forces.

We realized then that not only can we identify the goals of the system that the role reflects, but by implication we can also influence the originating system itself by weakening its restraining forces and thus influence the role-system vectors that are system outputs. By influencing the role-system through weakening restraining forces, we can also influence its relationship to inner-person system developmental goals. Thus, whenever one recognizes a role whose output will reflect the goal of the particular system that "sent it," not only can we identify the system that the role reflects but, by influencing the role-system (weakening its restraining force output), we can also influence the *goals* of the system itself. This was a brand-new understanding for us and quite exciting!

Back to our illustration of roles in our person-as-a-system

In our illustration (see Figure 4.1), the inner-person system roles have the potential for transferring energy/information between the survivor and the inner-person system, between the survivor and the explorer within the inner-person system, and across the boundary between the inner-person system and the inter-person system as well as the whole system and the hierarchy of systems.

These illustrations provided SCT a way of identifying the context for different therapeutic or organizational interventions by discriminating between the different goals in each of the three systems: the inner-person with the goal of survival, the inter-person with the goal of development, and the system-as-a-whole with the goal of transformation. In fact, these illustrations can be used by SCT practitioners to identify in which system context the roles are located: survivor or explorer inner-person role-systems, inter-person member (or subgroup) systems, or the underlying unlimited energy that fuels the system-as-a-whole.

Diagnosing the system that is the source of the role allows the SCT practitioner to recognize the resources the person in the role has available – both the resources of the role-system itself and the resources that are compatible with the context in which the role–system is functioning. Thus, the individual person's "freedom" to change depends not only upon their own resources but also on the resources available at the whole system level in the phase of development that is the current context. This is especially important in therapy where the whole system resources in the therapy system with its differential roles of client and therapist are the context for the client's inner- and inter-person change. Similarly, the whole system resources in a team determine what role-systems are driving and restraining.

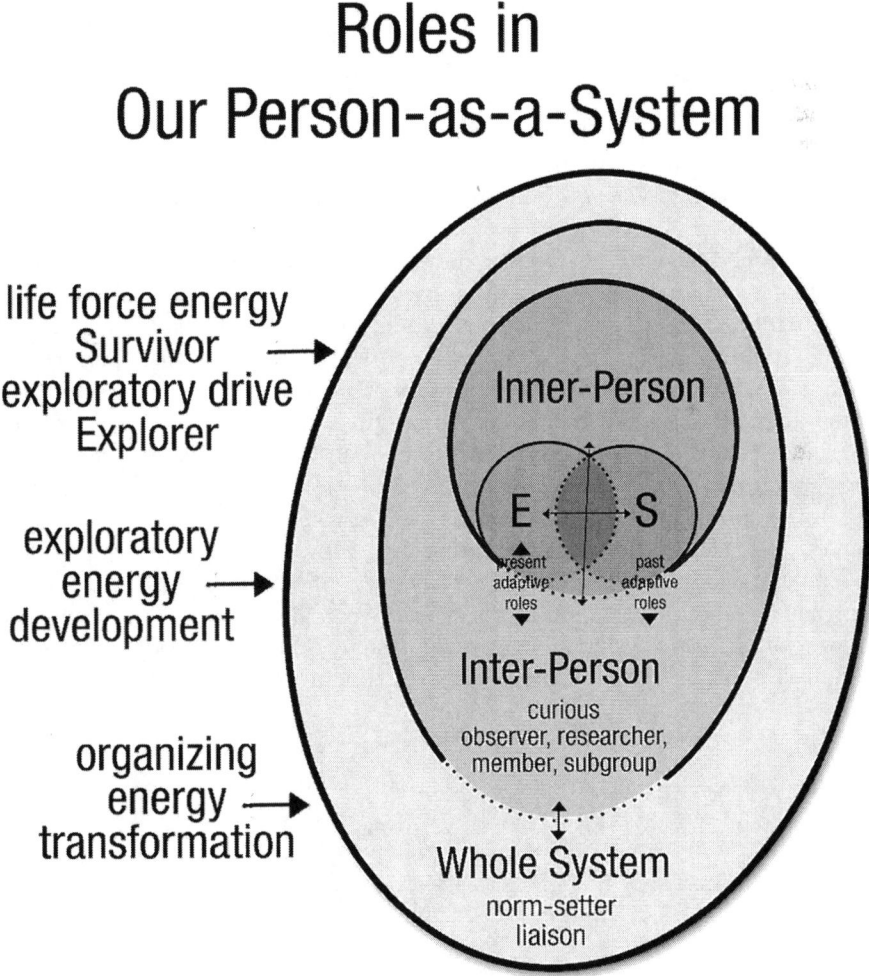

Roles in
Our Person-as-a-System

life force energy
Survivor ⟶
exploratory drive
Explorer

exploratory
energy ⟶
development

organizing
energy ⟶
transformation

Inner-Person

E ⟵⟶ S

present
adaptive
roles

past
adaptive
roles

Inter-Person

curious
observer, researcher,
member, subgroup

Whole System

norm-setter
liaison

Figure 4.1

"Roles" cross boundaries

One of the advantages in defining roles in terms of system dynamics is that the construct of role makes a useful bridge between SCT and the outside world. The word "role" links between the work in psychology and sociology, particularly the similarities between some of the methods and theory of systems-centered practice and family systems theory (Middelberg, 2006). On the one hand, roles have a defined meaning in systems language and, on the other, roles have both a professional and a popular meaning in the language of people. The word "role" also has meaning when applied to the different approaches to interventions in organizations where there is a strong emphasis on taking one's work role. This gives an expanded meaning to our understanding that "roles" cross boundaries. This takes us next to looking at role-systems as energy-organizing.

Energy-organizing: role-system boundaries organize system energy

Like any living human system, role-system boundaries organize system energy by opening and closing. When systems are stable, their boundaries are relatively impermeable. They are closed systems with a stable equilibrium oriented to the goal of survival. When the system is open, its boundaries can titrate, opening and closing according to the goal and context, and move towards developmental goals and close their boundaries to become closed systems when their stability is threatened.

Theoretically, the goal of all systems is to maintain a viable equilibrium. One way of so doing is by titrating boundary permeability. We know that when incompatible differences have crossed the boundary into the system, the "invaded" system develops subsystems to contain them. All can still go well if the system then works the process of discrimination and integration inside the system by joining on similarities and opening to small differences (the same process as successful functional subgrouping). However, when differences are too different for integration to take place, the difference is contained within impermeable boundaries, similar to an oyster containing an irritant within an encapsulating pearl. When the survivor system is under threat, it closes its boundaries and becomes a closed system (see Figure 4.7).

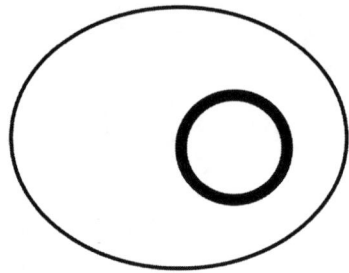

Figure 4.7

Systems close their boundaries when their survival is threatened. We have argued that system *survival* is at stake when differences are so different that they threaten to disrupt the internal equilibrium of the system. From a systems perspective, we "close" our boundaries to differences that would otherwise disrupt our functioning equilibrium and preserve our status quo: a driving force for system survival but a restraining force for system development! In our everyday world, all humans (and animals) react to differences as if they are a threat. Animals fight, flee or freeze at differences – and so do humans. In real life, we close our boundaries to ward off being "invaded" by others' opinions when they contain disruptive information that contradicts what we believe. Thus, a closed survivor role-system protects the life force from threats to its life force, and the open survivor role-system with its survivor boundaries opens to the curiosity of the exploratory drive, which is necessary if the survivor system is to develop and fuel development at all levels of the hierarchy.

Recapping, both open and closed systems have goals that are driving forces in relationship to one goal and restraining forces to the opposing goal. The open survivor system is a driving force to development. The inner-person "closed mind" of the personalizing role-systems is a driving force for survival even though unyielding and unchanging, in contrast to the open survival role-systems which maintain the potential for becoming.

This all translated well for us in developing our understanding of role-systems. SCT can now assume that whenever one recognizes a role, that role will be an output that reflects the goal of the originating system, so that we can decide in what way the role-system itself is a driving or restraining force in relationship to the system goal. For example, if the role is a personalizing or closed boundaried role, we can recognize that it is a driving force in closing inner-person survival system boundaries to a destabilizing threat. Recognizing this means that we can then reality-test the level of threat in the present. We can also see it as a restraining force to inner-person survivor system development.

Elaborating the idea of roles as role-systems is both a quantum leap in our theory as well as a significant new orientation in our SCT practice (this is elaborated in Chapter 5). Once again summarizing our theory, role-systems are defined, like all systems, as a hierarchy of isomorphic systems (similar in structure and function) that survive, develop and transform through discriminating and integrating differences and are goal-directing, energy-organizing, and self-correcting. We have so far discussed role-systems in terms of how they are goal-directing as well as how Lewin's (1951) work also served as a springboard for understanding more about how role-systems are energy-organizing. Our own explorations as described later in this chapter and in Chapters 5 and 6 show how a systems-centered perspective contributes to developing our inner- and inter-person human ability to self-correct roles from the past to respond to the goals of the present context.

Before exploring how role-systems are self-correcting, we want to visit some of the neurobiology that we have found helpful in our theorizing about energy and how energy is organized in our whole hierarchy of role-systems.

A detour to interpersonal neurobiology to help map role-system energy

We have strengthened our thinking about our role-systems by making a link between our theory of role-systems and their behavioral output and various neuroscience models that help formulate ideas about the energy that fuels our role-system behavior. The work of two members in our SCT community has been especially useful to us in integrating interpersonal neurobiology into SCT and being able to draw from neuroscience models in our theorizing about the person-as-a-system and the energy that fuels our person-as-a-system triad: that of Marianne Bentzen (Bentzen, 2015a, 2015b, 2018; Bentzen & Hart, 2015, 2018) and Susan Gantt (Gantt, 2018; Gantt & Agazarian, 2010, 2011; Gantt & Badenoch, 2013, 2020; Gantt & Cox, 2010). Their work, which is both similar to and different from each other's, has enabled us to draw from two different brain models to explore and expand our thinking about role-system theory. We start with Marianne Bentzen's work with the triune brain model that has helped us deepen our understanding of energy in our triad.

Seeing the energy in role-systems from the triune brain model

In discussions with Marianne, we made a connection between the energy that is organized in role-systems and the long-standing, popularized model of the triune brain (MacLean, 1990). Marianne Bentzen's (2015a, 2018) guides on neuro-affective personality development provide an illustrated elaboration of MacLean's triune brain model which itself has helped bring neuroscience into popular understanding. Marianne's illustrations of the triune brain model have been especially useful in distilling MacLean's model and in our learning how to think about ourselves and others through looking at how our brains work as well as in thinking about attunement and empathy.

The triune brain model is widely referred to in popular literature yet, as is true with any model or theory, the triune brain model has driving and restraining forces and in the scientific field is often criticized as an overly simplistic model and as out-of-date (it was originally developed in the 1960s) (King, 2017). In spite of its restraining forces, this model and modern tripartite derivatives of it are used in affective neuroscience (Montag & Davis, 2018; Panksepp, 2004; Sapolsky, 2017). We have found that its very simplicity and Marianne's translation of its broad brush strokes into everyday understandings have been helpful to us and our trainees in understanding intuitively how different brain organizations process human energy, enabling us to think more about energy in our theoretical triad of the person-as-a-system.

Briefly, MacLean's (1990) triune brain model identifies three "brain" systems. First is our instinctive *reptilian brain* centered in the brain stem, which can precipitate us into instant and automatic impulses to "flight, fight or freeze" when the experience of threat arises. However, with the experience of sufficient safety, this system also fuels curiosity and distinguishes degrees of pleasure or displeasure as well as the basic experiences of synchronized sensory interactions that form the foundations for complex emotional development. We see this as the source of our emotional social exploratory drive and our inherently rewarding curiosity about us and others. In contrast, our limbic system *mammalian brain* is our emotional brain and the source of our feelings and heartfelt resonance when we attune to other people or to our essential selves or to other mammals. This is the source of our ability to resonate with the feelings of others, participate in shared emotional processes and develop complex emotional interaction responses and roles, including empathic feelings. Our third brain region is our *primate brain* in our prefrontal cortex which allows us to *explain* and *test* our realities and consciously control and regulate our behavior as well as apprehend and intuit.

Applying this model to think about the different organizations of energy in our role-systems enables us to conceptualize our different levels of role-systems (inner-person, inter-person, whole system) as fueled by different brain systems as depicted in the triune model. We can see our inner-person system roles, fueled by the life force and the exploratory drive, as related more to the instinctive brain and our curious limbic system. We experience the sensory energy of the instinctive system as essentially a self-centered and self-focused life force where we automatically react with instinctive flight, fight or freeze responses when we feel our life force is threatened. These automatic responses occur when we experience danger in the present and can also occur from reacting from role-systems developed in the past to manage our conflicts with our significant others when we were suddenly "dropped." Our inter-person system roles, fueled by our curiosity and relationship to the goals of our context, are related more to our animal limbic and human prefrontal cortex as is our apprehensive, averbal experience.

Discovering our whole system knowing at the edge of the unknown

Apprehending our system-as-a-whole requires all of our brain energies: a sense that there is more to one's personal self than one is aware of in the moment; a sense that there is more to our inter-person relationships and to our inter-personal goal behaviors than can be explained; and a sense that there are levels of meaning that we may be able to intuit and which, over time, we can begin to define, like the whole system influence on our group and individual behavior of the phases of development of the group-as-a-whole. Our inner-person role-systems are fueled by our instinctive brain and limbic system. Our inter-person role-systems are fueled by both our limbic system and our prefrontal cortex. Our whole system role-systems come from an apprehensive awareness that is basically without words. SCT calls this sitting at the edge of the unknown.

"Sitting at the edge of the unknown" with curiosity is by no means easy! Apprehending our system-as-a-whole requires sitting at the edge of the unknown with curiosity in spite of our fear of not knowing. This is difficult for our human brain to do because all animals, and we are no exception, hate the challenge of the inevitable differences that exist within the vast areas of our unknowns at the same time as we are lured by our curiosity to explore them. Our human challenge is that sitting at the edge of the unknown is the source of new knowledge. In SCT we use the practice of centering (as described in Chapter 5) to access the energy at the edge of the unknown where there are no words!

As with all living human systems, role-systems survive, develop and transform from simpler to more complex when we discriminate and integrate differences. It perhaps goes without saying that for all of us, sitting at the edge of the unknown challenges us to be open to differences: differences that we must learn to tolerate if we are to discover what we don't yet know. It takes practice to sit at the edge of the unknown. Over time, in SCT, we can develop our ability to sit at the edge of the unknown, with curiosity, in spite of our natural fear of "not knowing."

Explaining as a restraining force to whole system knowing and exploring as a driving force for knowing the whole system unknown

Our human brain is a great explainer! As humans, we hate not only differences but also uncertainty, and one of the major differences that we all face every day is uncertainty (which is always a difference) about what is going to happen next. We hate uncertainty, and we all have the tendency to explain our future before we have lived it. We defend against the unknown by "explaining" it. Explaining bypasses our curiosity about our context with negative or positive predictions about the future which give us anxiety or hope from, respectively, our negative or positive feelings and shut out our curiosity and exploratory drive. We are also no longer in touch with our emotional and apprehensive sense of the world around us in the present which we can only be in touch with by exploring. From our neurobiological perspective, when we are in negative or positive predictions, we are using primarily our thinking human brain, our prefrontal cortex, and bypassing our feeling animal limbic system, where we can attune and resonate with ourselves, each other and our context.

Other inputs from interpersonal neurobiology

Susan Gantt has also worked for a number of years to integrate interpersonal neurobiology into SCT (Gantt, 2018; Gantt & Agazarian, 2010, 2011; Gantt & Badenoch, 2013, 2020; Gantt & Cox, 2010). Susan has drawn more from the brain model that sees our hemispheric brain as two brains in terms of function, or in a systems view, two internal subgroups. The right/left brain model has been deprecated for many years, yet this model of the brain has been newly re-embraced in interpersonal neurobiology fueled by the work of Iain McGilchrist (2009) and Allan Schore (2019). We have used these newer understandings of our dual brain processing systems, both our right and left brain, to deepen our understanding of inter-person relating. Susan's integration of this work has offered us a way to understand the differences in how human energy is processed dependent on whether it is right- or left-brain processing. For example, McGilchrist describes how each hemisphere "attends" differently and consequently "sees" and "experiences" a different world. In right brain processing, we focus on what happens between here-and-now emergence and flow. Further, Porges (1995, 2011) has demonstrated that our social engagement circuits are right-lateralized so that our social brain functions are more right-centric (Gantt & Badenoch, 2020). In contrast, our left brain organizes information into systems, puts pieces together and generalizes from data. As we elaborate in Chapter 6, Susan has concluded that the co-regulation that happens in the inter-person system enables greater and greater differentiation in right brain regulation capacity in the inner-person system. Further, building on the work of Schore (2010, 2012), Porges (1995, 2011), and Coan (Beckes & Coan, 2011; Coan, 2008; Coan & Sbarra, 2015), she has proposed that functional subgrouping (inter-person system) in particular develops our social brain functioning. Many in the interpersonal neurobiology field see the human brain as essentially a social brain (Cozolino, 2010, 2012, 2014) whose regulation is always primarily in co-regulation (Badenoch, 2011, 2017). Functional subgrouping both co-regulates energy and develops our co-regulating right brain function. Similarly, it is in co-regulating with others that we feel secure and most easily open to curiosity and can more easily bear the unknown and the implicit, wordless unknown that our right brain intuits.

Both of these models of brain function that Marianne and Susan have introduced to SCT have been useful for us thinking about energy in our person system hierarchy and in deepening our understanding of our human challenges of learning to stay curious at the edge of the unknown. This work in integrating interpersonal neurobiology into SCT has enabled us to revisit an important theoretical question about the edge of the unknown.

Curiosity at the edge of the unknown

The theoretical question that arises at the edge of the unknown is "what is the source of the universal knowledge that exists for us before we have words to explain it?" And why does it arouse annihilating anxiety rather than wonder?

Our system-as-a-whole goal of intuitive understanding without words is related to our capacity to sit at the edge of the unknown and gradually intuit meaning out of the underlying chaos that exists in all systems. It is related to understanding system isomorphy (similar to "parallel process"). It is also the threshold of discovering the "selfless self," which experiences the world without words before it can translate it into human meaning.

SCT suggests that the "unknown" is the source of the universal knowledge – the threshold between knowing and not knowing that exists for us before we have words to explain it. For each of us, this is at the brink of chaos. Chaos can easily arouse our fear with our flight, fight or freeze responses. As Porges (1995, 2011) has demonstrated, we have no control over our instinctive responses when we experience threats to survival or, as we say in SCT, our boundaries just close; we don't close them, they close us. Our autonomic nervous system reacts instinctively. In contrast, our curiosity is fueled by our exploratory drive, staying curious at the edge of the unknown before "explaining" the future requires us to "sit at the edge of the unknown," an experience that arouses a combination of curiosity and fear and is more easily borne in the co-regulating experience of subgrouping functionally (Gantt, 2018). When we are dominated by our flight/fight responses in our reptilian brain, we can no longer grapple with the challenges of connecting to our averbal experiences at the edge of the unknown and our right brain apprehension of the bigger picture. Instead, we can only do our best to survive. Our more threatening freeze responses range from terror to annihilation anxiety, all of which dominates our experience at the cost of the unknown which is infinitely different.

The responses to threat in our survival system are also present in many systems of the worlds we live in. We are thus often puppets on the strings of the current phase of development of our context, without any awareness that it is not simply our own dynamics that are influencing our experience. As we will see in Chapters 8 and 9, which focus on phases of system development, not only are we not the only pebble on the beach, but it is the beach in interaction with the tides of the sea that has the greatest impact on the shape of the pebble that is our self!

Our explorations of interpersonal neurobiology helped us to deepen our understanding of energy and how we process energy/information. Seeing role-systems as goal-directing and energy-organizing was rich for us and laid an important platform for returning to in our newer illustrations as we consider how role-systems are self-correcting.

Self-correcting

Our new illustrations have helped us understand more about self-correcting in our person system. We start by revisiting our person-as-self or our emerging inner-person system to explore how the potential for self-correction is inherent in our inner-person and in our inter-person and our person-as-a-whole role-systems.

Self-correcting: our survivor and explorer role-systems in our emerging inner-person system

Our closed boundaried survivor role-system keeps out differences (see Figure 4.8), yet our TLHS says that any living human system survives, develops and transforms by discriminating and integrating differences.

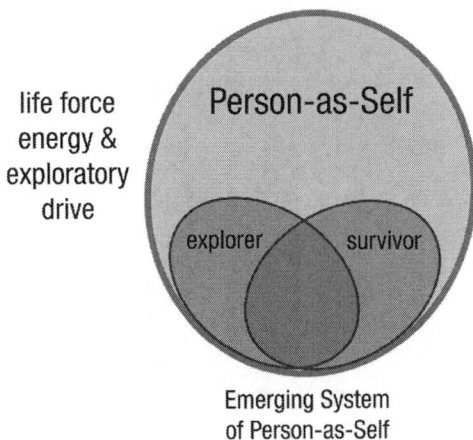

Figure 4.8

In order to develop and transform, survivor system boundaries need to be appropriately permeable to the exploratory drive (see Figure 4.9). This requires being open to our explorer system with its available curiosity!

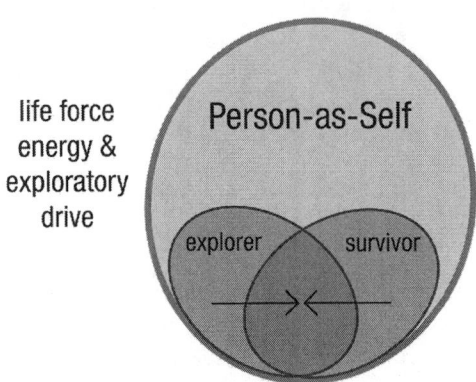

Figure 4.9

When we are curious, our boundaries are permeable and we can move towards our developmental goals (see Figure 4.10). When we are not curious, our reality-testing fails and our exploratory drive, which fuels self-correction, is no longer available.

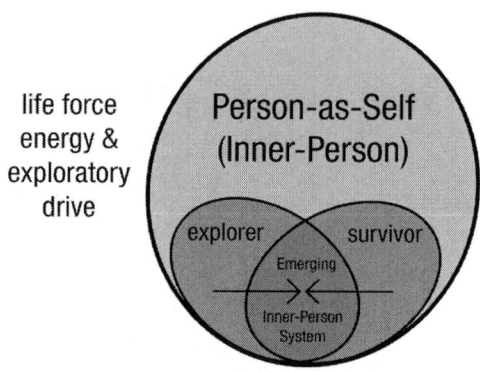

Figure 4.10

The three previous figures (4.8, 4.9, 4.10) illustrate the interchange between the survivor system with permeable boundaries and the curious explorer system. When we are curious, our explorer boundaries open and we attune to our survivor role rather than reacting in a way that threatens it and closes its boundary. We can think of this as our explorer subgroup and survivor subgroup integrating, or our explorer joining the survivor subgroup and bringing in the small difference of curiosity. This implements self-correcting in our inner-person system.

Both open and closed systems have goals that are driving forces in relationship to one goal and restraining forces to the opposing goal. The open survivor system is a driving force to development. The inner-person "closed mind" of the personalizing role-systems is a driving force for survival in the known, firmly unyielding and unchanging. This contrasts with the open survival role-systems, which maintain the potential for becoming and developing in the unknown.

We need both subjective person-centered apprehension and our exploratory drive with our curiosity about our experience of our inside self and our experience of the world around us. When we are curious, we can connect our life force energy to our exploration of what we are curious about. When we are not curious, we are connected to just ourselves. To our astonishment, we had discovered that curiosity is a criterion that differentiated between person and personalizing, or open or closed survivor roles.

The life force and exploratory drive

As we introduce in Chapter 5, both the life force and the exploratory drive are necessary if systems are to survive and develop and transform. Survival depends upon the energy of the life force and is necessary for the survival of the hierarchy. Development depends upon the energy of the exploratory drive. Both are necessary for the development of every system in the hierarchy. Thus, both energies are necessary and neither one is sufficient alone.

Discriminating and integrating differences

From our SCT perspective, there are two kinds of differences that all living human systems (including role-systems) need to integrate in order to survive, develop and transform: differences in the apparently similar and similarities in the apparently different. It is a fundamental assumption in SCT that increasing one's ability to discriminate and integrate differences is not only *necessary* but also *sufficient* for reaching the goals of all successful change processes, including therapy! Thus, the inner-person contains both the life force which provides the energy for survival and the exploratory drive which provides the energy for change. The overall goal of the inner-person is system survival by discriminating and integrating its different energies, life force *and* exploratory drive, as a surviving, developing and transforming survival system. The goal of the inter-person system is system development and to relate to the goals of the context, and the goal of the whole system is to contain and transform system norms. Our inner, self-aware self relates to the energy of our inner self in contrast to the energy that relates inter-personally with others. Inter-personal systems are dependent on the context, and membership is related to the goals of the context. Each system is its own context as a surviving, developing and transforming system and each system has a role in the system hierarchy.

Our companion illustration (see Figure 4.11) further illustrates the avenues of self-correction: first for releasing the development potential within the inner-person system and then the potential for transferring inner-person role-system development across the boundary into the inter-person context.

Importantly, the inter-person context in subgrouping creates a secure context for exploring, similar to what Porges (2011) calls social engagement. Subgrouping facilitates neuroception of safety in which our boundaries can open to small differences in the context of the similarity of being understood. Functional subgrouping is also an essential self-correcting system as it facilitates boundaries opening to small differences in the context of similarities. This enables integrating differences, supporting self-correction towards the interdependent goals of survival, development and transformation. Functional subgrouping also supports what Porges has identified as our human preference for connection for regulation instead of flight or fight which orients us to survivor roles. This is also how functional subgrouping then makes a self-correcting and self-potentiating system of development at all system levels, where the inter-person subgrouping supports development in the explorer which can then

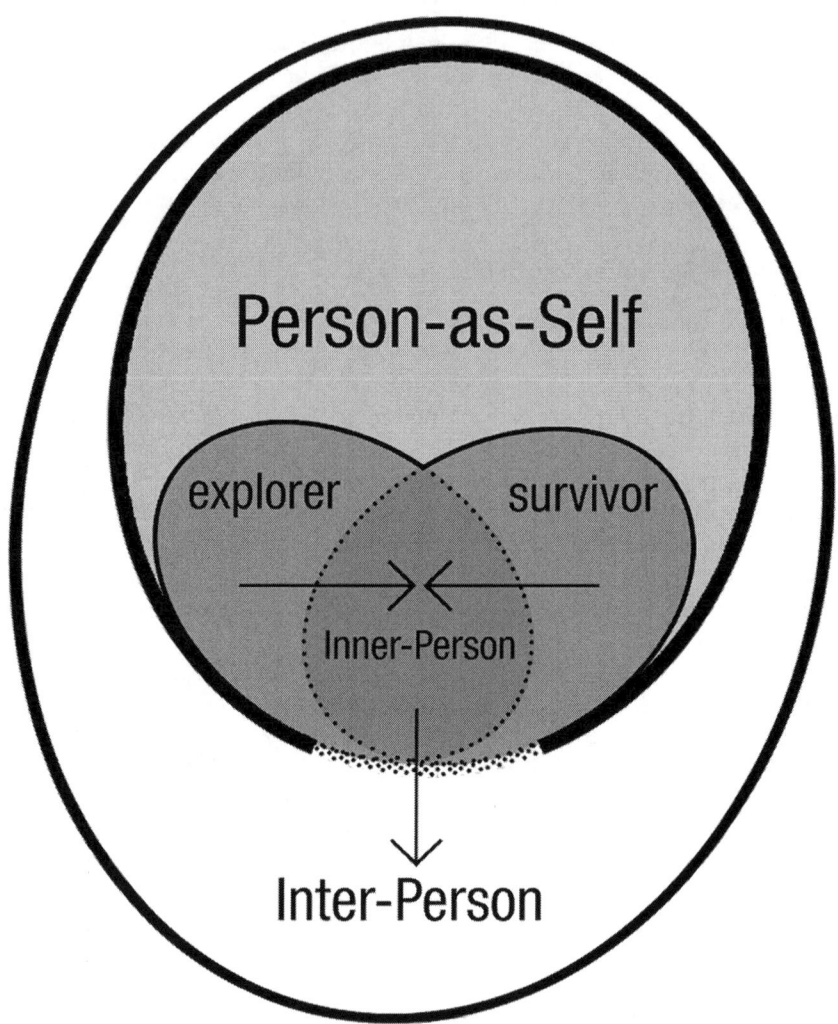

Figure 4.11

transfer across the boundary to the survivor system and potentially fuel inner-person system development as well (refer again to Figure 4.1). The subgrouping systems discriminate and integrate the differences which then influence the norms and transformation of the whole system. Importantly, as the group system develops, the subgrouping process increasingly develops the implicit right to right brain communications that Schore (2019) sees as the heart of psychotherapy.

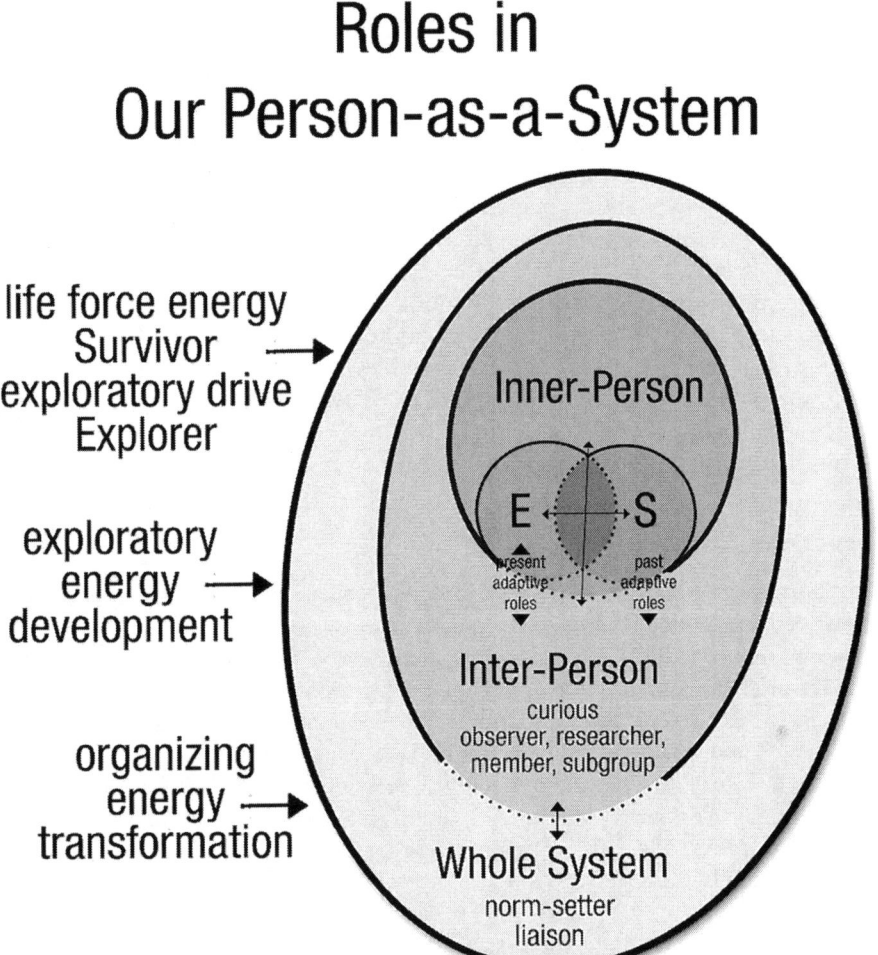

Roles in
Our Person-as-a-System

life force energy
Survivor
exploratory drive
Explorer

exploratory
energy
development

organizing
energy
transformation

Inner-Person

E ⟷ S

present
adaptive
roles

past
adaptive
roles

Inter-Person
curious
observer, researcher,
member, subgroup

Whole System
norm-setter
liaison

Figure 4.1

Past adaptive roles

Our past adaptive roles first develop in our survivor system under two different conditions: threat and no threat. When our survivor system is not under threat, our boundaries are potentially permeable to the curiosity roles of our explorer system with access to the exploratory drive as well as the life force. These are our primary person roles, whose development potential is limited only by context dynamics. The other set of roles, our closed survivor roles, are past adaptive roles developed in response to threat from differences or conflicts over differences.

Developing survivor roles in the past under threat

SCT discriminates between role-systems developed in the past and role-systems developed in the present. Past role-systems developed in the context of the past to manage differences and challenges in the past. These roles are related more to the past than the present. They are actually out of context when they are imported into the present and repeat in the present what was a role-system solution that belongs to the past. We also call these closed roles "secondary person" roles. They respond to perceived threats with flight, fight or freeze roles. These survivor roles are often activated in the present when the survivor system experiences threat, either triggered by universal signals (like a blank face) or someone not behind their eyes or by look-a-like present role inductions that mirror the past or by the phase of the system's development. Threats don't come out of the blue. They have two sources: inside us or outside ourselves. When something in the present reminds us of our past, we can retreat into the same old roles that "saved" us in the past. When we do this, we are rarely conscious that we have literally retreated from the present into a past adaptation.

Repetition compulsion roles

Our inner-person survival system roles are fueled by life force energy and originally developed as a driving force in protecting our innate sense of self. Past adaptive roles are comfortably familiar (a driving force). However, their boundaries are mostly closed to differences in the present. They are the source of our repetition compulsions and, thus, they are also a restraining force. Originally developed as an interface between us and our significant others and essential to our survival and emotional security, these roles import the past into the present where they are out of context. We call these roles our repetition compulsion roles. These closed survival roles are relatively impermeable to any differences and instead only open to the comfortably apparently similar, and they are the source of stereotyped subgrouping.

Past roles are rarely useful in the present as they are out of context as the goals of the roles belong to the past, not the present. These repetition compulsion roles repeat in the present the solutions that we developed in the past to frustrations. Though these roles were adaptive in the past when first developed, past adaptive roles are out of context when imported into the present. Past role-systems elicit past role-system responses, and before one knows it, one's experience is governed by the repetition compulsion, a system of closed interactive role-systems.

Present adaptive roles

What is similar (and new) is the idea that all roles when they were originally developed are adaptive. What is different is discriminating in the present whether a role originates in the past or in the present. We can distinguish past roles from present roles by identifying the context and goals of the role. Role-systems developed in the present develop in relationship to the context and goals of the present, whereas past roles have already developed within a different context with different goals. Past adaptive roles interface at the boundary between the survivor and the inter-person system, fueled by the life force. Present adaptive roles are at the boundary between the explorer and the inter-person system and are fueled by the exploratory drive. This recognition has had significant impact on the practice of SCT, which we elaborate in Chapter 6.

Illustration: role-systems at the boundaries

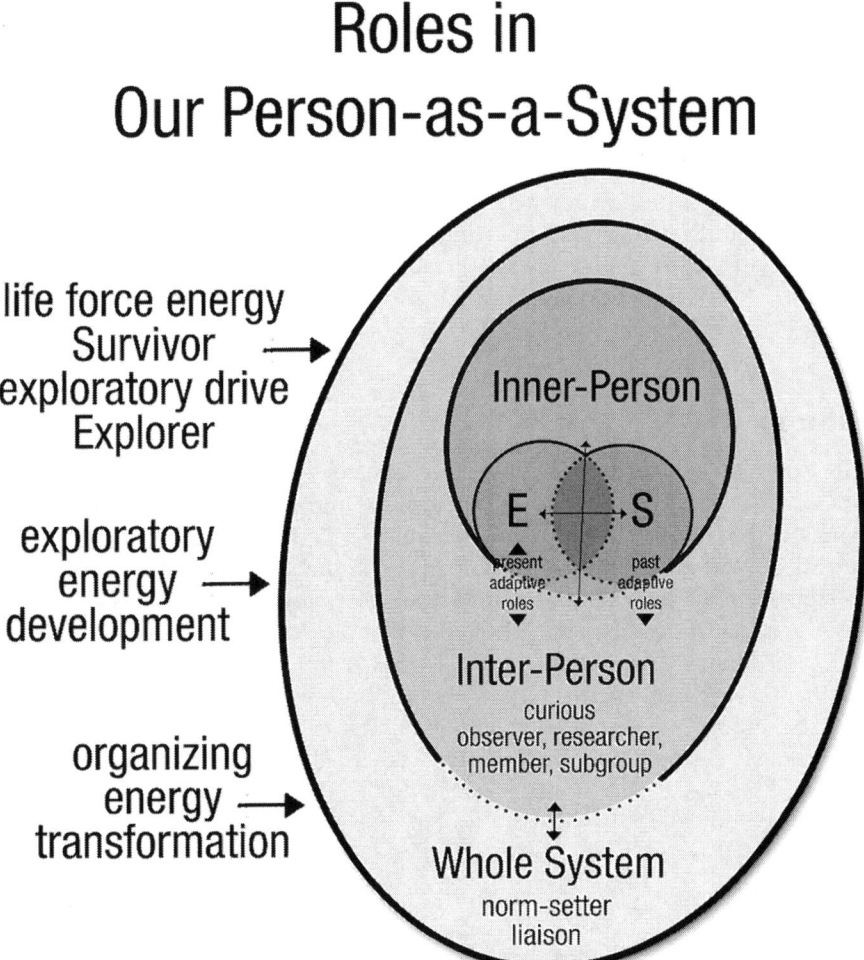

Roles in Our Person-as-a-System

Figure 4.1

Revisiting this illustration (see Figure 4.1), we can now use this illustration to help us identify role-systems at the boundaries both within and between systems. We can define role-systems as containing the energy/information necessary for system survival, development and transformation. We have allocated past adaptive and present adaptive roles to different subsystems in the inner-person system. Past adaptive roles are fueled by and protect the life force. These past roles are at the boundary between the survivor and the inter-person system. In contrast, the present adaptive roles are fueled by the exploratory drive and are at the boundary between the explorer and the inter-person system roles developed in the present in relationship to the goals of the present, whereas past roles have already been developed within a different context with different goals.

We emphasize that all roles are adaptive when first developed. This frees us from thinking about roles in terms of pathology and instead relates them to the context of past or present. This is probably one of the basic contributions of SCT: understanding that all so-called "defenses" are driving forces in titrating the boundaries of the inner-person survival system so that the system can maintain an equilibrium when threatened by differences that are too different to be integrated without de-differentiating. In other words, defenses are neg-entropic responses to entropic threats. Thus, early role-systems are always adaptive when first developed yet are out of context when imported into the present!

Summary

Energy emerges from the inner-person survivor system and is fueled by the exploratory drive. The energy/information from the inner-person system then crosses its boundaries to our inter-person system, where it is organized with its goal of maturation and transformation. The inter-person system goal is to develop by integrating the communications that cross its boundaries.

We have introduced the idea of role-systems which are characterized by the isomorphic dynamics of all systems in a defined hierarchy. Role-systems are then energy-organizing, goal-directing and self-correcting. The energy they contain is the energy/information that is transferred across the boundaries between systems, specifically from the sending system to the receiving system. This has a new implication for SCT: that the goals of the sending system are conveyed by role-systems. The response from the receiving system is determined by its goals. Importantly, defining roles as systems has added the dimension of isomorphy to our definition of roles as vectors, which our original definition of vectors did not have. All systems are isomorphic: similar in structure and function but different in different contexts. For example, we can think about how role-system boundaries are all potentially permeable, but when they close or open will depend upon the relationship between the energy/information contained within the role that is a function of the "sending" system and its compatibility to the energy/information within the "receiving" system. For example: someone relating to their sense of self (inner-person survivor system role) will let in only compatible responses and close to differences, whereas someone relating inter-personally can remain curious about differences (inter-person researcher system role) and has the potential to take a role with others in the subgrouping and explore and process "differences" for the system-as-a-whole. Thus role-system interactions can serve as driving or restraining forces for the survival, development and transformation of the system-as-a-whole context: both the differences in the apparently similar and the similarities in the apparently different.

Seeing the role-systems at the boundary is also useful to highlight one of the major differences between systems-centered therapy and many other orientations: in SCT, the major change interventions are directed more to the *inter-person* system than to either the *inner-person* system or the *person-system-as-a-whole*. This is based on the assumption that, because of its common boundaries with the *inner-person* and *person-system-as-a-whole*, the therapeutic changes in the *inter-person* member system have the greatest potential for influencing change in all three. Thus, the focus in systems-centered therapy is consistently to increase the capacity to discriminate and integrate differences in every middle system in the hierarchy, with the expectation that this one intervention will increase the probability of the survival, development and transformation of the whole system hierarchy. Our next two chapters present how we are taking our new role-system theory into SCT practice.

References

Agazarian, Y. M. (1992, February). *The use of two observation systems to analyze the communication patterns in two videotapes of the interpersonal approach to group psychotherapy.* [Based on I. D. Yalom "Understanding group psychotherapy" (videotape). Pacific Grove, CA: Brooks-Cole]. Panel on "Contrasting views of representative group events", American Group Psychotherapy Association Annual Meeting, New Orleans, LA, US.

Agazarian, Y. M., & Peters, R. (1981). *The visible and invisible group.* London, UK: Routledge & Kegan Paul. Reprinted in paperback (1987). London, UK: Karnac Books.

Badenoch, B. (2011). *The brain-savvy therapist's workbook.* New York, NY: Norton.

Badenoch, B. (2017). *The heart of trauma: Healing the embodied brain in the context of relationships (Norton series on interpersonal neurobiology).* New York, NY: Norton.

Beckes, L., & Coan, J. A. (2011). Social baseline theory: The role of social proximity in emotion and economy of action. *Social and Personality Psychology Compass, 5*(12), 976–988. doi:10.1080/10926771.2013.813882

Bentzen, M. (2015a). *The neuroaffective picture book.* Rothersthorpe, UK: Paragon Publishing.

Bentzen, M. (2015b). Dances of connection: Neuroaffective development in clinical work with attachment. *Body, Movement and Dance in Psychotherapy, 10*(4), 211–226. doi:10.1080/17432979.2015.1064479

Bentzen, M. (2018). *The neuroaffective picture book: An illustrated introduction to developmental neuropsychology.* Berkeley, CA: North Atlantic Books.

Bentzen, M., & Hart, S. (2015). *Through windows of opportunity: A neuroaffective approach to child psychotherapy.* London, UK: Karnac Books.

Bentzen, M., & Hart, S. (2018). *The neuroaffective picture book 2: Socialization and personality.* Rothersthorpe, UK: Paragon Publishing.

Coan, J. A. (2008). Toward a neuroscience of attachment. In J. Cassidy & P. R. Shaver (Eds.), *Handbook of attachment: Theory, research, and clinical implications* (2nd ed., pp. 241–265). New York, NY: Guilford Press.

Coan, J. A., & Sbarra, D. A. (2015). Social baseline theory: The social regulation of risk and effort. *Current Opinion in Psychology, 1,* 87–91. doi:10.1016/j.copsyc.2014.12.021

Cozolino, L. (2010). *The neuroscience of psychotherapy: Healing the social brain* (2nd ed.). New York, NY: Norton.

Cozolino, L. (2012). *The neuroscience of psychotherapy: Building and rebuilding the human brain* (2nd ed.). New York, NY: Norton.

Cozolino, L. (2014). *The neuroscience of human relationships: Attachment and the developing social brain.* New York, NY: Norton.

Gantt, S. P. (2018). Developing groups that change our minds and transform our brains: Systems-centered's functional subgrouping, its impact on our neurobiology, and its role in each phase of group development. *Psychoanalytic Inquiry: Today's Bridge between Psychoanalysis and the Group World [Special Issue], 38*(4), 270–284. doi:10.1080/07351690.2018.1444851

Gantt, S. P., & Agazarian, Y. M. (2010). Developing the group mind through functional subgrouping: Linking systems-centered training (SCT) and interpersonal neurobiology. *International Journal of Group Psychotherapy, 60*(4), 515–544. doi:10.1521/ijgp.2010.60.4.515

Gantt, S. P., & Agazarian, Y. M. (2011). The group mind, systems-centred functional subgrouping, and interpersonal neurobiology. In E. Hopper & H. Weinberg (Eds.), *The social unconscious in persons, groups, and societies: Volume 1: Mainly theory* (pp. 99–123). London, UK: Karnac Books.

Gantt, S. P., & Badenoch, B. (Eds.). (2013). *The interpersonal neurobiology of group psychotherapy and group process.* London, UK: Karnac Books.

Gantt, S. P., & Badenoch, B. (2020). Systems-centered group psychotherapy: Developing a group mind that supports right brain function and right-left-right hemispheric integration. In R. Tweedy (Ed.), *The divided therapist: Hemispheric difference and contemporary psychotherapy.* London, UK: Routledge.

Gantt, S. P., & Cox, P. (Eds.). (2010). Introduction to the special issue: Neurobiology and building interpersonal systems: Groups, couples, and beyond [special issue]. *International Journal of Group Psychotherapy, 60*(4), 455–460. doi:10.1521/ijgp.2010.60.4.455

King, P. (2017, August 10). *What is the current scientific status of the triune brain theory proposed by MacLean?* Retrieved from www.quora.com/What-is-the-current-scientific-status-of-the-triune-brain-theory-proposed-by-MacLean

Lewin, K. (1951). *Field theory in social science.* New York, NY: Harper & Row.

MacLean, P. D. (1990). *The triune brain in evolution: Role in paleocerebral functions.* New York, NY: Springer Science & Business Media.

McGilchrist, I. (2009). *The master and his emissary: The divided brain and the making of the western world.* New Haven, CT and London, UK: Yale University Press.

Middelberg, C. (2006). When the group is really a family: Application of systems-centered therapy techniques to family therapy. In S. P. Gantt & Y. M. Agazarian (Eds.),

Systems-centered therapy: In clinical practice with individuals, families and groups (pp. 144–163). Livermore, CA: WingSpan Press. Reprint (2011). London, UK: Karnac Books.

Montag, C., & Davis, K. L. (2018). Affective neuroscience theory and personality: An update. *Personality Neuroscience, 1*(e12), 1–12. doi:10.1017/ pen.2018.10

Panksepp, J. (2004). *Affective neuroscience: The foundations of human and animal emotions.* New York, NY: Oxford University Press.

Porges, S. W. (1995). Orienting in a defensive world: Mammalian modifications of our evolutionary heritage: A polyvagal theory. *Psychophysiology, 32*(4), 301–318. doi:10.1111/j.1469-8986.1995.tb01213.x

Porges, S. W. (2011). *The polyvagal theory: Neurophysiological foundations of emotions, attachment, communication, and self-regulation.* New York, NY: Norton.

Sapolsky, R. M. (2017). *Behave: The biology of humans at our best and worst.* London, UK: Penguin Books.

Schore, A. N. (2010). The right brain implicit self: A central mechanism of the psychotherapy change process. In J. Petrucelli (Ed.), *Knowing, not-knowing and sort-of-knowing: Psychoanalysis and the experience of uncertainty* (pp. 177–202). London, UK: Karnac Books.

Schore, A. N. (2012). *The science of the art of psychotherapy.* New York, NY: Norton.

Schore, A. N. (2019). *Right brain psychotherapy.* New York, NY: Norton.

Simon, A., & Agazarian, Y. M. (1967). *SAVI: Sequential analysis of verbal interaction.* Philadelphia, PA: Research for Better Schools.

Chapter 5

Role-systems in systems-centered practice

As we have discussed, defining roles as role-systems and as system outputs enabled us to see that each role-system contains the same goals as their originating system. We can then observe in the everyday world whether the goals of our role-systems, that we can now identify, are received or rejected by their target system. In other words, when is each specific role-system a driving or restraining force in the process of transferring the energy/information that they contain to another system? And how do we assess this?

Putting our role-systems map into practice

Focusing on the dynamics of the roles that we play has been implicit in much of our earlier work. For many years, we have been familiar with roles that emerged within groups, stimulated by the phases of system development, like the roles of identified patient and scapegoat (Agazarian & Peters, 1981). We had also long recognized that system-as-a-whole phase dynamics were a more powerful influence on how we take up our roles than our own free choice. Yet before our new illustrations and newer theory with its focus on the person-as-a-system, we had not yet understood how truly important it is to see a role as related to its context in our person system.

Expanding the application of our theory to include roles as systems led us to discover not only new implications from our theory but also new methods for our systems-centered practice, including insights into the development of our early survivor roles (see Figure 5.1). Most importantly, we are now more deeply understanding that however self-defeating or antisocial our roles can be, understanding them from a systems framework is less likely to arouse the hatred or shame that all too often occurs when we separate our past relationships into "good" and "bad" (our human pull to splitting).

Roles in
Our Person-as-a-System

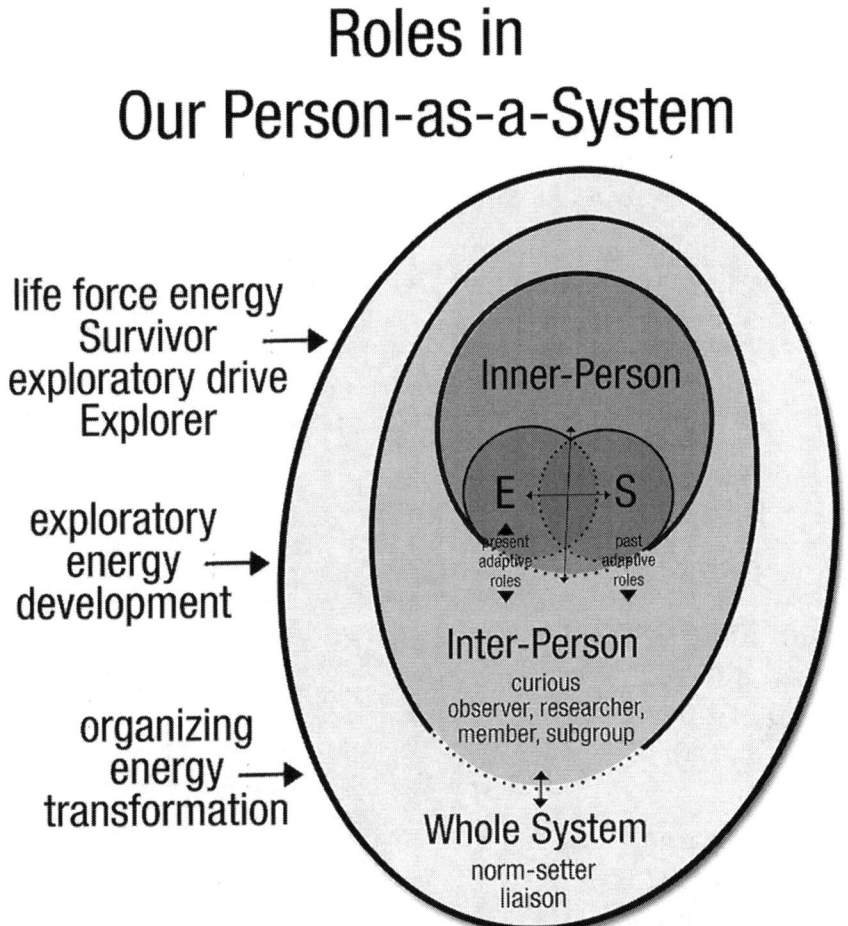

Figure 5.1

Role-systems and goals in the real world

When we are exploring our own responses to our context, we are fueled by our inner-person role-systems with their life force and exploratory drive. In contrast, when we are subgrouping functionally, we are in our inter-person fueled by our life force and exploratory drive and our inter-person roles. The goals of how our energy is used change as we shift from the inner-person goals of survival and development to our inter-personal goals of our development in context with others. This nicely integrates and extends our original SCT saying of "role, goal and context," which we can now apply in this case to how our goals change and our roles change as our system context changes from inner-person to inter-person systems to whole-system roles! This leads us to exploring our person-as-a-system illustration as a map to guide us in our every-day life as people, therapists, consultants and managers to be better able to take up our role, goal and context in all areas of our life.

Exploring our roles in our person-as-a-system

Locating roles in the system context they represent led us to discover that our new illustration (see Figure 5.2) is useful in recognizing which of the three systems to which we are related at any moment in time. We can identify our role-system as belonging to one of our three systems: inner-person, inter-person

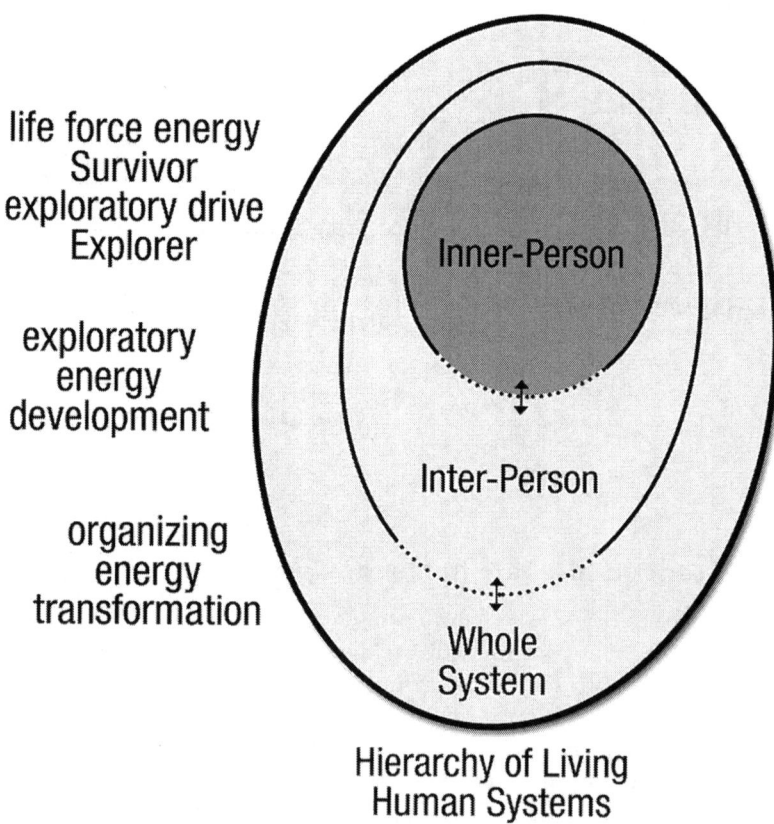

Our Person-as-a-System

life force energy
Survivor
exploratory drive
Explorer

exploratory
energy
development

organizing
energy
transformation

Inner-Person

Inter-Person

Whole
System

Hierarchy of Living
Human Systems

Figure 5.2

or system-as-a-whole. As each system has its own characteristic roles, this lets us know where we are by the role we are in! And each of the three systems has a different goal, quite useful in that we can again use the SCT mantra of "role, goal, context" to orient us to *mindfully* choose the role that supports the goal of our context. In short, we discovered that our illustration can be used as a map. The illustration above is the simplest of our maps. As you will have seen in our illustrations in the preceding chapters, our role-systems "maps" also have developed from simpler to more complex. In this, our simpler map, we begin with how we have used these illustrations to map our role-systems and then discuss how mapping our role-systems has revolutionized our systems-centered practice.

If we look at Figure 5.2 again, we can see it differently by thinking of it as a map that allows us to locate the system in which our roles originate. By locating the systems from which our role originates, we can also identify our system goals as each region of the map has a specific system goal. What makes using our illustration as a map particularly useful for systems-centered practitioners is that, as we discussed in Chapter 4, the goals of our role-systems will always be the same as the goals of the system that "breeds" them, once again building on Lewin (1951). Thus, by observing and identifying our roles, we can tell the system in which we are living and to which of our three system goals we are relating: survival, development or transformation.

The goals of all inner-person role-systems will relate to survival and orient towards the primary inner-person system: the survival and development of one's essential self. For example, if we want to work towards our goals for personal growth, we want to develop our inner-person role-systems. In contrast, our inter-person system goals relate to development and to working with others or alone towards social goals in our environment. If we want to develop our skills in working with others towards mutual goals, we develop our inter-person role-systems. The goals of our whole system relate to transformation and will reflect the whole system dynamics at all levels of the hierarchy, like the phase of system development, the maintenance of operational norms, relating to larger contexts still and transformations of universal systems for better or worse. Black holes probably swallow each other! If we want to better understand the unseen influence of the different levels in the hierarchy of the system-as-a whole, we want to develop our role-system for sitting at the edge of the unknown.

Identifying where we are on the map by the way we talk

Serendipity! It was at this point in our work on defining roles that our work from the 1960s in defining SAVI (Simon & Agazarian, 1967) again held us in good stead as background. Returning to SAVI enabled us to operationally define role-systems as having system outputs that are recognizable by the way we talk (more on this in Chapters 7 and 8). As we introduced in Chapter 2, Shannon and Weaver (1964) had theorized that ambiguity and redundancy were "noise" and that "noise" as they defined it was entropic to the transfer of information in a communication channel. Noise is like static on our phones that makes it hard to hear the speaker. Simon and Agazarian added contradiction as a third source of noise in human communication. This was quite useful to link with our burgeoning understanding of role-systems and their outputs in that we recognized that any time a communication was ambiguous, contradictory or redundant, it indicated a closed boundaried role-system.

The next step was to see how to identify when our goals as reflected in our verbal communications belonged to our inner-person, our inter-person or our whole person. In Chapter 4, we described how role-systems are outputs from their system of origin. Building on this understanding, we recognized that we have three different languages, one for the inner-person system, another for the inter-person system and still another for our system-as-a-whole. What is more, each of our "output" behaviors signals which of our three systems is sending them.

Recognizing our inner-person system language

"Inner-person system language" identifies us as being in the context of the first person (with "I" or "my" or "I know or think or feel . . ."). It is fitting that we first called our inner-person our "person-as-self." We are mostly interested in ourselves and less interested in others or our context! In our inner-person system, we use the language of introspection: "I" language. We talk about "me" and "my" thoughts and "my" feelings. Our voice tone and our gestures and body postures match our self-centered communication as we talk about ourselves. We are often not behind our eyes, or we are primarily watching to see whether the other (or others) is listening to us! These behavioral signals are easy to identify in ourselves and others once we have learned to recognize them.

Returning to our illustration (Figure 5.1), it is useful to remember that we have available to us two different role subsystems in our inner-person system with two different energies (life force energy and exploratory drive). These energies fuel our inner-person goal of being met as a person, and when we are, we are gratified in our person system survival. When we close our boundaries in a fixed role, we have no choice except to personalize our person system. We will tend to take everything "just personally" as our goal is only inner-person survival. If we are in attuned resonance with others and met as a person, we are satisfied. In contrast, it is painful or enraging when we are not.

Our inner-person system with its roles and energies is then reflected in how we talk. If we are also curious about how we are taking things personally, we can ask ourselves "what role am I in?" By so doing, we can explicitly take note about how we are "talking" signals the system we are in and the goal we have at that moment: whether our "talk" is related mostly to inner-person goals or inter-person goals or, as we will discuss later in this chapter, whether we have been induced by others' roles or the context (or are inducting others) into a role lock.

Roles in
Our Person-as-a-System

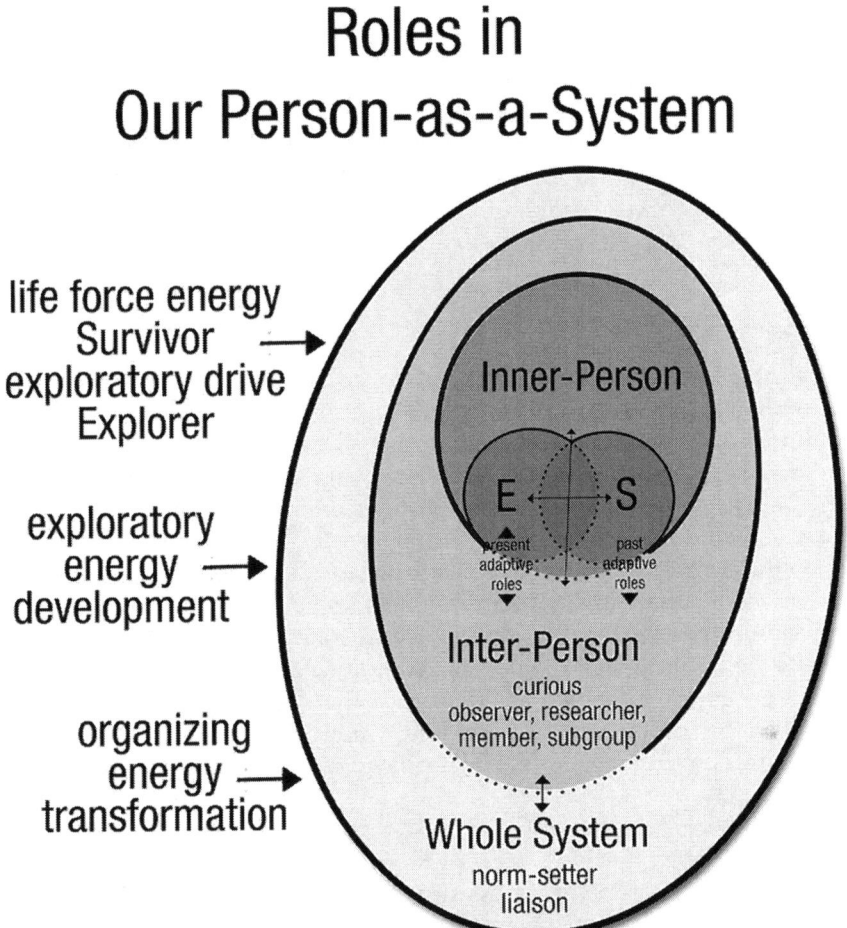

life force energy
Survivor
exploratory drive
Explorer

exploratory
energy
development

organizing
energy
transformation

Inner-Person

E   S

present
adaptive
roles

past
adaptive
roles

Inter-Person
curious
observer, researcher,
member, subgroup

Whole System
norm-setter
liaison

Figure 5.1

Curiosity and our inner-person exploratory drive

Whether we have a choice to explore our inner-person roles depends upon whether we have access to our exploratory drive. When we are curious, we have access to our inner-person exploratory drive. When we have closed our boundary to our exploratory drive, we have retreated into our closed survival subsystems. Whether we are curious will be reflected in both what we say and how we say it. For example, if we are judging our survivor role ("it is really stupid that I do that"), there is no curiosity or exploratory drive. In contrast, phrases like "I am really interested in . . ." or "I am curious . . ." signal that our exploratory drive is active.

Closed survivor system

In our closed survivor role-system, we have closed our minds, have closed our boundaries to all outside influences and have cut off from ourselves as a whole person and from our personal context. When our curiosity fails, we are helplessly in the grips of our repetition compulsion, repeating past roles that *were* adaptive when they were first developed but are impermeable to change in the present. Our "talk" when we are in this system is full of "yes, but" or "no" or "not me" or "not how it is for me" or "I'm right, and you are wrong" or even denial, and we stubbornly hang onto where we are in this role as if that is our only way to survive.

Narcissism

We can roughly equate the life force in the core person system with primary narcissism. We can also equate the roles that develop as mediators between the core life force survival system and the demands of our care-takers with secondary narcissism. When in our secondary narcissism roles, we are fiercely protective of our hard-won compromises and fight off any attempts to modify our behavior. We take every difference just personally. Taking everything personally, on the one hand, uses the role that was originally developed to protect our primary life force (the driving force). On the other hand, it prevents us from reality-testing and negotiating with the world around us (the restraining force). We have no curiosity when we personalize, just a fierce resistance to anything that is different from the way we see it and often visible in a language pattern of "yes, but" or explanation. Survival is not enough; we must also develop, and in order to develop we must be able to negotiate the differences between us and the outside world.

In our inner-person survival roles which involve personalizing from a self-absorbed self-centeredness, we have an expectation that others should please us. This leads us to positive expectations of others. The reverse is other-centered personalizing in which one is absorbed in pleasing others who will then be completely pleased and satisfied. In SCT, these roles typically surface in the authority phase of development.

Negative expectations arise from our inner-person survival roles when they involve self-absorption around negativity, personal pain and an expectation that no help or understanding exists. Or we can be absorbed in others' negativity or pain with the expectation that we will be overwhelmed by it. In SCT, these roles are worked with in the intimacy phase of system development.

Locating our role-system on the map will tell us where we are and "who" we are, both by how we talk and also by observing the way we behave in our role! For example, if we are focusing on our self-development with curiosity, we are in a "developing" inner-person role that can lead to personal insight. If we have the same inner-person focus without curiosity, we are in our "closed" survivor role, safe from any personal insights! Thus, when we personalize, we cannot use the exploratory drive we were also born with. We are all born with both a life force and an exploratory drive so that within our inner-person system we have both energies available to us unless we are personalizing and become dominated by the repetition compulsion.

Recognizing our inter-person system language

It is not difficult to "recognize" the shift from our inner-person self to the self that is open to others, that is our inter-person system. It is our inter-personal self that is aware of both others and our real-world context. We will hear ourselves say "I and you, or we . . ." or "Oh look at . . ." or "Do you know? feel? want? think?" or "Shall we?"

In SCT, the best and most obvious example of our inter-personal language is the language of functional subgrouping. In functional subgrouping, we use the discipline of "reflection" before we build on others' ideas. This requires reflecting the other person before one responds. In reflecting, we join others with a reflection of what they have communicated until they know and "feel" that they have been heard and understood. When it is our turn, we alert others when we have finished our input by saying "anyone else?" Functional subgrouping ensures the goal of communication has been met. It provides data about whether information has been transferred from the talking person to the listening person. Functional subgrouping is "functional" in that it prevents the "parallel talk" that sounds "as if" a conversation is going on when very little information is getting across! Most important of all, functional subgrouping, as Chapters 1 and 2 describe, enables any living human system to more easily integrate differences and function to survive, develop, and transform. It may go without saying that SCT's functional subgrouping has introduced a new way of working towards the goals of the inter-personal system.

We can also call the inter-person the "we" system with its shared goals. This contrasts with the inner-person goals in the system of "me." The whole system influences "we" and "me," and "me" and "we" fuel the whole system. Inter-person goals are the development of mutual goals, and whenever we are working with others towards (or away from) different goals, we are located in our inter-person system (see Figure 5.3).

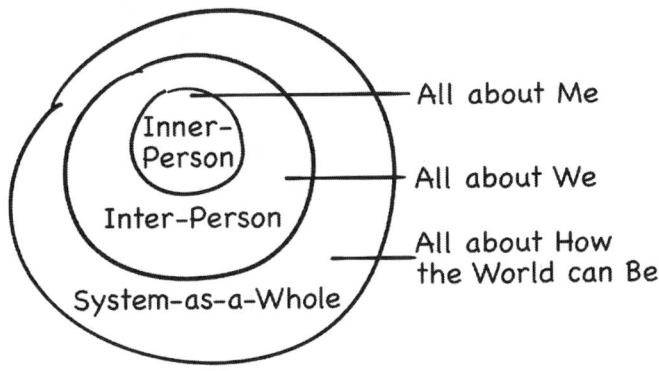

Figure 5.3

The language of our whole system

If we are involved in whole system development, we are involved in the many levels of goals in the system hierarchy. Recognizing the whole system communications is not so easy because we depend upon a meta-level of awareness to notice them. The whole system influence is like an unseen intervening variable that casts a shadow between the system-as-a-whole and the role-systems that are elicited. Citing the "elephant-in-the-room," for example, is a familiar way of expressing the "feeling" that there are unseen influences at work, when we are not quite sure what it is we are intuiting! We can though, for example, become aware of role-system behaviors that seem to be marching to a different drum from any that we can hear. It is what we mean in SCT when we say every person is a voice for themselves and also a voice for the group-as-a-whole. Or as we often say: each of us are puppets on the strings of group dynamics.

From our SCT work on phases of system development (see Chapters 8 and 9), we now take it for granted that when the group elects the role-system of the all-too-familiar group identified patient, the whole system of the group is in the flight phase and when the group induces the role-system of scapegoat, the whole system has shifted into a fight phase. Identified patients or scapegoats are good examples of role-systems in the phases of whole system development that are elicited respectively in the flight and fight phases. So are the compliant or defiant roles that are the hallmark of authority role-system relationships. So also are the merging or alienated role-systems elicited in the phase of intimacy. Recognizing these and crossing the boundary into an awareness of the whole system influence in the present gives us the potential to choose to transfer into work role-systems in the present. Parenthetically, it is only when we can diagnose the whole system goals of the moment that we can think about whether the identified patient or scapegoat role-system is a driving or restraining force! In SCT, we call this underlying whole system dynamic a system projective identification. It is also known as parallel process.

In summary, by recognizing our "talk" and our behaviors, we can recognize our role-systems. If we recognize our role-system, we can recognize where we are on our map: whether we are "living" in our inner-person system, our inter-person system or whole system. By looking at the illustrations and using them as a map to identify ourselves in a specific system, we can see whether the system in which we are located is relevant to our goals and to our contexts and, if not, see what we will have to do to change if we wish to cross the boundaries into another system.

Differences among psychodynamic, cognitive and systems-centered therapy

There is a significant difference between SCT and psychodynamic therapy when it assigns all present problems to our childhood without recognizing the impact of other dynamics of the various systems that influenced our childhood and continue to influence our everyday lives. This leads us to a fundamental difference between SCT and most psychodynamic and cognitive therapies: SCT introduces the implicit influence of the many systems-as-a-whole on how we develop our roles and on the process and outcome of therapeutic practice. This is particularly important to us as therapists, recognizing the parallels and role inductions between the many contexts that influence the therapy in the present, inside and outside the case room. We are rarely specifically aware, for example, that every therapist's office serves as the context for system dynamics that influence both patients and therapists in individual therapy, couples therapy, family therapy or groups. There are also other invisible influences of the context, like the norms of the systems, private practice, clinic, hospital, mental health organization and our country and its laws and norms. From the perspective of system isomorphy and hierarchy, all of these systems will have an invisible impact on the therapeutic process. We can then see the past as one of the contexts rather than a cause!

When we enter a therapeutic situation, whether as a therapist or a patient, the first important boundary to cross is between being our self as a person and becoming a member of the context. In SCT therapy, it is through our experiences as a member that our person system changes in the direction of the therapeutic goals. This is true for both the therapist and the patient. Strangely enough, thinking about patients as systems can make it more likely to treat patients like people. In SCT, there is always a therapeutic neutrality but also a human connection in the methods which requires working together with empathy and attunement with the three different role-systems of a person. Another advantage of thinking about people in terms of the three systems is that SCT assumes that unless our changes reach the core center of ourselves (our central inner-person system fueled by the life force), the changes that we make will be confined to what we think and what we do but will not be changes in our essential inner-person system, which is where our core sense of identity is contained. In other words, change comes not from explaining but from experiencing so that change can then be integrated into our core self.

Seeing one's role in context rather than taking one's role just personally

It is important not to take our roles just personally! Roles are not the person. Locating oneself on our map has provided great relief when our members recognize that their role behavior belongs to the system, not the person. Seeing roles as systems opened the door to understanding that roles do not exist in a vacuum. They exist in context. Inner-person roles exist in the inner-person context, inter-person roles exist in the inter-person context, and whole system roles exist in the system-as-a-whole.

Also importantly, our role-systems did not develop in a vacuum – they developed as part of interactive systems in the past in the context of early care-seeking and socializing influences with others. In reality, we know we cannot possibly be in an ideal relationship all the time, much as we want it. Thus, when there are compromises to be made, when our significant other's responses to us have more to do with them than us, we develop useful, compromise role-systems. These role-systems mediate between our instinctive knowing of the attunement and resonance that is "right" for us and the compromises we must make to get as much of what we want as is possible in the real world. Similarly, our ongoing challenge is how best to contribute to the world to which we belong so that it develops and, in turn, develops us!

An important focus for therapy is to discriminate whether a closed role is an import from the past or whether it is a response to the present context, where we want to keep our differences and protect our system equilibrium. Stabilizing our equilibrium is a useful response in the short run. Making this discrimination in the present as to when we do need to stabilize, or when we do not, is essential so that we can learn to assess both when and when not to protect our system equilibrium by closing our boundaries. Mapping our role-systems helps normalize and de-pathologize our role-systems, making it more likely that we can assess when or when not to retreat to a closed role.

Our focus on mapping role-systems has also proved useful in organizational coaching and team and leadership development (Gantt, 2013). For example, our role-systems map has been a useful guide both to support inter-person or member orientation to role, goal and context and to learn to weaken the restraining forces that prevent one from taking one's role in context.

Using our map to see our roles in context has deepened our understanding not only that roles do not exist without a context but also that they have an impact on others' roles in our inter-person context. Our role communications induce others to reciprocate from their roles, and the result is a role lock system which governs us and them both and can only be changed when the role lock is understood as a system. Before we elaborate on role inductions and role locks, we visit role behaviors and postures that, like our "talk," signal our role-system and its context.

Role postures

Just as our verbal behavior and language indicate our role-system, our nonverbal behavior is also a major indicator of our role-system and goals. All roles can be identified by their postures. Connecting how our postures change when we shift from one region on our map to another is a useful way of linking our behavior to the roles. Our roles reflect the "output" of the system in which we are located. Just as with our "talk," we can link the role postures that signal role-systems to the different regions on our map, and we can also assume that our role-system goals have the same goals as their sponsoring system. We therefore can intuit, by observing the role-system behavior, whether they are driving or restraining forces in relationship to our current goals!

It is relatively easy to become aware of role postures and connect them to the role that is expressing the system that the person is experiencing. Inner-person role

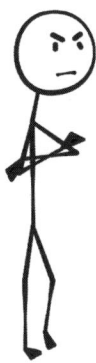

Figure 5.4

postures signal that the person is basically related to themselves (e.g., looking up signals relating to one's "thinking" role or stubbornly closing to protect oneself [see Figure 5.4]), and personalizing role postures (e.g., a flat face) are different from personal attuned role postures (e.g., responsive face). Each tends to induce different role responses from others. It is from open systems in our inner-person selves that we relate to others with resonance and attunement.

Further, in SCT we actively discourage past adaptive role postures in our here-and-now work and in our relationships when the posture reinforces early role adaptations at the cost of present role adaptations. Not only do we actively work to stop ourselves and others from sitting in role postures that tend to induce reciprocal roles in others, we also encourage both ourselves and others to undo role postures by beginning every work session with the "centering exercise," summarized here:

> Sit comfortably, feel the support of our chair and the floor under our feet. Become aware of our breathing, in and out. As we breathe out, follow our breath down, deeply into our center. Where we know without words. From our centered connection with ourselves, bringing our energy into our member role and gaze around the group.

The goal is to have our life force and exploratory curiosity available for work, rather than compromised as happens when we retreat into old adaptive roles. By finding alternatives to our old roles, we are free to respond with roles that are adaptive in the present, whether our present is in our inner-person system, our inter-person system or our system-as-a-whole.

Role postures will also signal the driving and restraining forces that let us know how ready our patients are for work. For example, we discourage depressed patients from sitting slumped, which reinforces their feelings of hopelessness and a role lock with the self. Similarly, an SCT group that is sitting slumped in silence is manifestly not ready to work. In contrast, a group that is silent but alert or that is actively subgrouping in resonant communication will appear attentive and centered with plenty of available energy. This leads us next to role inductions and role locks that impact the inter-person system.

Role inductions and role locks

Our behaviors are outputs from role postures. These role postures developed as part of our roles in the past as we negotiated our way through our developmental phases and now get reproduced (and potentially modified) in the present. What is sometimes less obvious is that role postures tend to induce reciprocal role postures – and if we are not aware of the role induction, before we know it, we have been induced into a role response, which can easily end up as a role lock. In a role lock, the output of your survivor role induces my survivor role and vice versa – this makes a very stable system. Sitting with legs crossed and head tilted up or looking down one's nose will probably elicit either competitive or submissive roles in others. Compliant postures of looking up and across from under one's eyebrows with one's head tilted down will probably elicit either care-taking or dismissive role responses. Or one-up can elicit a one-down reciprocal role or defiant role and vice versa (see Figure 5.5).

Role inductions

We define "role induction" as our experience of being pulled to role by responding to another person's role behaviors from a reciprocal role in ourselves. We often unwittingly enact our role inductions with others. SCT sees

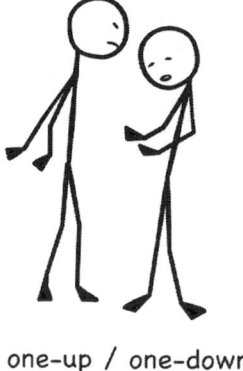   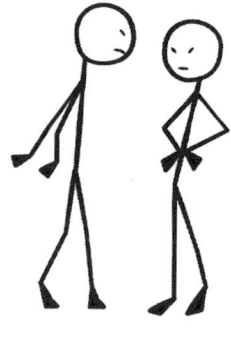

one-up / one-down   one-up / defiant

Figure 5.5

this phenomenon as a major influence on how we have spontaneous reactions to a mismatch between others' roles and our own. We react to the difference, and the shock of the mismatch between us and the other is easily experienced as personal. When we are in a here–and–now relationship, we are likely to adapt to these mismatches, using our past roles that we originally developed to manage the "shock" of the loss of the relationship in our early mismatches. In our past, mismatches occurred in our very early experiences when we were in an attuned attachment relationship with our significant others and we were suddenly "dropped." This same distress is replicated in our present responses when we regress into the past roles that we developed to manage the loss of affiliative attachments when we were very young, for example, when the "other" disappears into themselves and personalizes.

It is only through recognizing and exploring role inductions in the present that we come to notice that we are often unknowingly reacting to the role signals that others send when they themselves retreat into past, personalized roles. On our side, we are often just as unaware that we are sending role signals ourselves. It takes curiosity about our inner-person selves to re-experience the present, and it also takes curiosity about our relationships (inter-person) to undo our role locks that are induced by role postures in the present.

In SCT, it has been helpful to discover that we will automatically react to the role signals sent by ourselves and others whether we "want" to or not. Our automatic reactions are fueled by the energy of our instinctive brain at the autonomic nervous system level. As Porges (1995, 2007, 2009, 2011) has demonstrated, being in connection with others is our preferred nervous system state when the other person's face is responsive to us. In contrast, in response to the loss of the affiliative connections between us and others (our animal limbic connections), our autonomic nervous system stabilizes in flight, fight or freeze. We can also be triggered when there are differences with others between our understandings of reality that are rooted in our human and prefrontal cortex. This is how we get pulled into role locks without understanding why. We have barely met the person and already we love or hate them!

Until we understand the inductive power of roles, we will not distinguish role locks as "relationships" fueled by the past which make us blind to role interactions in the present. In role locks, both of us are victims of our repetition compulsions. Unwittingly, retreating into our old roles tends to awaken reciprocal old roles in others, and we then become imprisoned in role locks which do, realistically, threaten our present. In role locks, we take things just personally and tend to close our boundaries to curiosity. Without curiosity about either ourselves or others, we tend to make "as if" relationships. In groups, we develop "as if" subgroups.

In contrast, fueled by our inner explorer, we can take up our inter-person observer and researcher roles and develop an awareness of threats that we react to without knowing. We can notice that we are implicitly reacting to the role signals that others send when they themselves retreat into past, personalized roles. Until we come to recognize the role signals sent by ourselves and others, we will automatically react to them and others will react to ours and transfer a past template onto a present person!

Interestingly, a role induction can be a driving or a restraining force. The difference is whether we are induced to respond from roles that we developed in the past to manage threats to our sense of self or whether we are induced into reciprocal roles that are in the service of here-and-now problem-solving. Once again, it is a relief when we recognize that role induction is a system property and not personal. Early roles were originally adaptive compromises that maintained our connection to our attachment relationships. If mother wanted it tidy, developing a tidy role enabled both to have pleasure even though the role comes at the cost of our own impulses. This is a good example of the challenges and successes in socialization.

Conscious and unconscious role inductions

There are some important realities over which we have no control. For example, as illuminated by Porges' (1995, 2007, 2009, 2011) work, we can think of our social brain as checking to see whether we are "safe" with others. That is, we are hardwired to open to others when they are responsive to us and just as strongly, to react to others when they do not appear friendly. Met with a blank face, our autonomic nervous system responds with flight or fight and we retreat into the survivor roles which helped us manage past losses of attunement and empathy! When we are not aware of these inductions, we are likely to be catapulted into an old reciprocal role-system or propel others into their old role-systems because we are not attuned to them. When we are relating to people who are unresponsive to us, or too different from us, it is easy for us to take it personally. When we take others just personally, we tend to respond with some of our old survivor roles, roles that often reciprocally match theirs, and then we get into a role lock. If we don't take it personally, we can always respond with our social selves. We can even have a good social time. However, a good social time is not the same as a deeply satisfying relationship when we are attuned with each other.

How our training groups discovered role locks as a system

One of the most productive changes in our training groups came as members developed the curiosity about the clues that enabled them to identify their own and each other's roles. These were ongoing groups and much of their group life was characteristic of the work phase. Guided by our new theory, group members could both support and be supported by an objective (inter-person) exploration into the clues that signaled role inductions as well as role locks. As members explored their reactions in our training groups, we made exciting discoveries of how old roles not only repeat the past but also serve as role inductions in the present. Seeing how our role posture induces reciprocal role postures was exciting. When we were not aware of the role induction, and really before we knew it, we were induced into a role response which could easily end up as a role lock. It was a great discovery for the whole group when members recognized that their role behavior induced others to reciprocate from their past roles. This led to the recognition that the result is a role lock *system* that governs them both and can only be changed when it is understood as a *system* that needs to change.

Our training groups were also excited as we discovered how to become aware when we have responded inside an old role and how we can become curious and discover the early adaptive roles that we developed. When we do this, we can observe the difference between the past and the present. We can then become curious about how to attune to the other whose role behavior is a trigger for us. We can get curious about the current context that is stimulating past role adaptations in both of us and in the group and, above all, we can learn how not to take either our own or others' role behavior just personally.

In continuing to apply our new theory, some training group members discovered even earlier roles that developed to manage experiences of misattunements and loss of mirroring. With continued exploration, they identified an experience of sensing nonverbal threat. At this level, their reactions included threats to their sense of self, which some understood as related to early failures in attunement and mirroring, quite important work in the training of therapists. It was through these explorations that we were able to recognize the difference between affiliation/attachment role development and social role development, which we will discuss in more detail in our next chapter.

Blank face

It was also in our training groups that we first explored the role inductions in response to a blank face. Using the systems-centered method of functional subgrouping as a container for their work, our training group members explored their own role responses to the blank face. For many members, their first spontaneous line of defense was to respond with whatever roles they had originally developed to manage their innate experience of distrust: for some it was the nonverbal experience of suspicion, and for others it was explanations of why they felt the other was misattuned to them. Some blamed the other, and some blamed themselves. All in all, the groups discovered that a blank face tended to elicit the roles related to flight or fight or sometimes freeze. Some group members even discovered how their own blank face was an output from their early survivor roles. Interestingly enough, the groups discovered that all of these roles were not only childhood solutions but also included roles that also related to later phases of development.

Again, these discoveries fit well with Porges' (1995, 2007, 2009, 2011) polyvagal theory where he identifies a hierarchy of autonomic nervous system responses with a human bias towards ventral vagal with its priority of connection to others: we look first to see whether the other is relating to us or is "there," so to speak. In SCT, this is from our inter-person. Drawing from Porges, if we "neurocept" danger instead of safety, our sympathetic nervous system activates and responds with flight or fight (signaling inner-person survivor roles). If we do not see a way out of danger, our dorsal vagal "freeze" takes over.

Interestingly, Tavistock group leaders often employ a blank face, which elicits early survivor role adaptations and often enactments of the survivor roles. Though this is often stressful for participants, the Tavistock training provides highly useful learnings. Similarly, when working with the authority issue in SCT, the leader often uses a neutral face to give the group greater freedom to project and discover their authority roles. Doing this work in the context of functional subgrouping lowers the stress of the survivor responses that are triggered and supports exploring in the inter-person context to discover information from the survivor roles in the context of authority.

Couples therapy and role locks

Couples therapy is a good example of working with a role locked system in that couples typically seek therapy when their role-system interactions are not working for them. It is frequently characteristic of both partners to be locked in roles that repeat the personal family dynamics of their pasts which they blame on each other as "character flaws"!

What tends to occur all too often in couples therapy is that the couple system establishes its role locks based on the repetition compulsion roles that each member system contributes. This implies that change in the dyadic couple system (the middle inter-person system) is the first step to enabling change in the person systems – and not the other way around in spite of couples often saying that the goal they have is for their partner to change! SCT introduces functional subgrouping to the couple as central to the process of influencing the norms of the couple system in that it invites inter-personal communication from attuned person systems. It has been an innovation in the practice of SCT couples counseling to recognize that the different functional role-systems that contain the couple are dyadic systems-as-a-whole: for example, the parenting role-system, the business role-system, the intimacy role-system, the person-to-person role-system and the developing system-as-a-whole, all of which take both of them to change (Agazarian & Gantt, 2014).

Using the person-as-a-system map with couples in undoing role locks

Our newer theory and map are proving highly useful in our work with couples. It provides a map for them to use that supports their recognizing when their conflicts are between various inter-person role-systems and the challenge of negotiating priorities or between the different roles in their inner-person or inter-person system or related to whole system norms. For example, one couple was in conflict over who was meant to pick up their daughter from school. It started when the wife, who was originally scheduled to pick up their daughter, asked the husband to pick her up from school. This looked initially like an inter-person role renegotiation over who was going to implement that parenting-role job that day. Using the role-systems map enabled us to see that their difficulty was over the unacknowledged change in their whole system family norm. It was an important norm for them as a family system to not change a plan that was set, and changing who was picking up the daughter was undoing an original plan. Significantly, the wife grew up in a family that never stuck to what they planned and so she made the proposal from a past adaptive role more related to her family of origin roles than to their present family norms. The couple had previously worked hard together to establish their family norms different from the ones she and he grew up with. Both of them wanted that for themselves and their daughter. Once the two of them could see it as a change in family norms, it was much easier to decide whether to change on this occasion as a practical adaptation or hold their norms together.

Using our new map as a role-systems map

In our explorations, we recognized that all of the work on roles in our person-as-a-system applies to all living human systems. Viewing our picture from this understanding, our illustrations can be used as role-systems maps that can be used to map ourselves as a person in all of our contexts and to map any whole system context. With this awareness, we added another version of our picture which orients us to using our more complex illustrations and expands it to use in any system hierarchy, and we called it a role-systems map (see Figure 5.6).

"Mapping" our roles rather than "repeating" old roles

This approach of mapping our role-systems has been useful in a range of contexts, whether it is for training or therapy or personal growth or coaching or team or leadership development. Learning to recognize or "map" our old roles has been enormously helpful to us and to our patients and clients and trainees. How the role-systems map is used is, of course different in different contexts.

When we are relating to someone and we are both in our inter-personal selves and the other then responds to us from their inner-person, we immediately feel dropped! In reality, what has been dropped is the limbic system resonance that had been between us. If we are aware of what has happened to us, we have the potential for avoiding a regression into our past adaptive roles that

Role-Systems Map

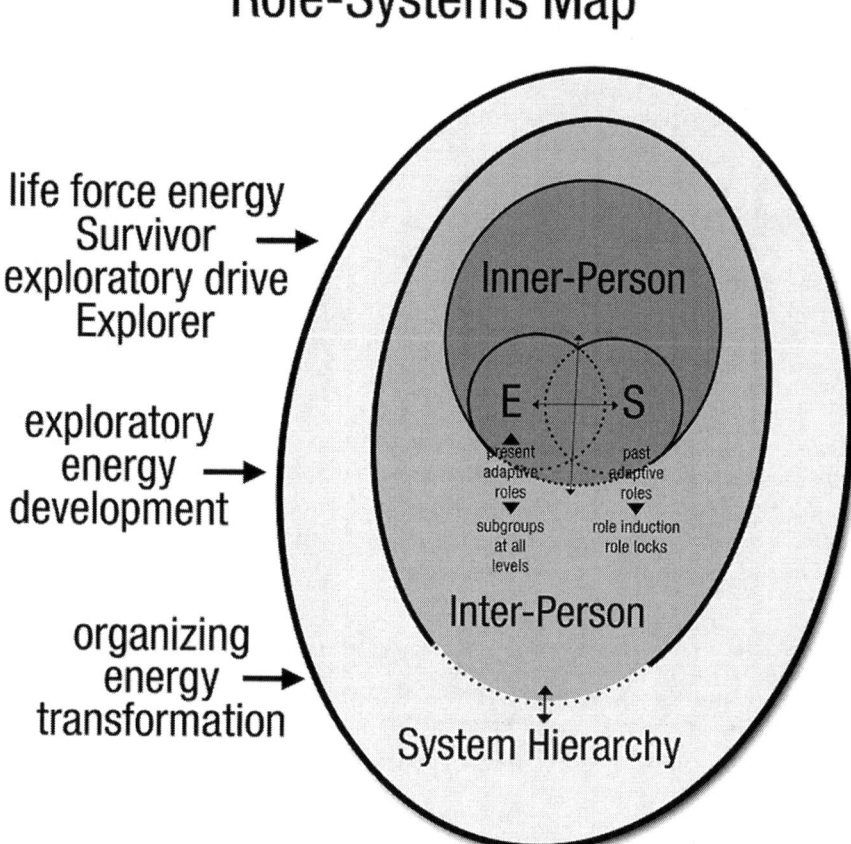

life force energy
Survivor →
exploratory drive
Explorer

exploratory
energy →
development

organizing
energy →
transformation

Inner-Person

E ← → S

present
adaptive
roles

past
adaptive
roles

subgroups
at all
levels

role induction
role locks

Inter-Person

System Hierarchy

Figure 5.6

managed earlier "drops" and which we developed to contain what we experience as a threat to our survival. Often, however, we are not even aware of the signals in the role shift between us and another. In this case, if we are unaware that we have been dropped, we automatically respond with our instinctive flight response into our early past adaptive role. Old roles worked in the past to manage what is for everyone a mini (or a maxi) trauma. However, as we know, old roles don't work for us in the present. Thus, past roles essential in past survival not only induce past experience but, because there is no longer present resonance or attunement when we are in a past role, tend to induce survival responses in others to losses of attunement in the present. Early in systems-centered therapy, there is less focus on how non-adaptive repetition compulsion roles developed in the past and more focus on how to restore access to here-and-now roles that can adapt to the present. Present drops require present adaptive roles.

Our map is useful in learning whether our role-systems are past or present (see Figure 5.6). If we are personalizing our experience (closed boundaries) and out of touch with our whole self, or scaring our self with look-alikes in our past (re-experiencing being anxious and tense and not sure how to behave or with impulses to disappear like we did then), then we are in role-systems that we developed in the past. Past role-systems are rarely useful in the present as the present is experienced "as if" it is the same as the past and, in past roles, we are closed to seeing how the present is different from the past. Our role relationships are experienced "as if" they are mirrors of the originals, and we tend to react the way we reacted then. When we experience the present as if it is the past, then we know we have retreated into old "closed secondary survivor role-systems" that we developed to protect our self and our relationships when we felt insecure and alone with no one to turn to but ourselves.

If we are able to activate our curiosity, we can recognize what has happened. This may be when our map is most useful. We can use our map and identify which system we are living in, decide which system we want to be in, and discover how to personally change both our system context and our role. If we are able to cross the boundary between our inner-person and our inter-person, we can join others so that we don't have to work all alone. In SCT, we can always look for a subgroup!

For example, when our feelings get hurt and we take everything personally, we can assume that we are relating from our inner-person system in our survivor subsystem and that the part of our survival that is under threat is our self-image and our goal is to defend it. If we become curious about our reactions, we have shifted from exclusively subjective experience, which often has no words, to include objective experience, which allows us to think. We can then assume we are relating from our curious explorer system, and our role behaviors will look and feel different from our hurt-feelings reactions. (We have also changed the potential for resolution. If we then start looking at the context [our explorer and researcher roles] and noticing that we were both tired and somewhat crabby [our researcher role collecting data], this indicates that we have crossed the boundary into our inter-person system.) Outputs and inputs from one system to another, and the impact of role inductions, both within individual people and between people at many different levels, are a fundamental challenge in all therapies and deliberately addressed in SCT. From this perspective, all role-systems are designed to serve as role inductions. Whether they are a role induction that is useful to the goals of the therapy system itself (or even a work team) can be judged by whether it is a driving or restraining force in relationship to the system goals.

Questions to guide our mapping

When we are in our personal-past with no personal-present, we are without curiosity and in a closed survivor role-system. One way we can tell which role-system we are in is by asking our self these questions:

Am I curious?
Am I in my inner-person self?
Am I in my personal inner-person self and shutting out others?

If so, I know I have not yet crossed into the inter-person system and am still in my inner-person past role-systems which I have imported into the present.

When we are in a personal-present role, we are in our curious survivor role-system. We can also identify this by asking questions that locate us:

Am I relating from my inner-person survivor with my boundaries open to roles that are appropriate to me, in relationship to the goals of the specific context with others?

Or am I unaware that the whole system context is inducing me into roles that relate to its whole system goals, whether or not I want to be in these roles or to support the whole system when the whole system is in fight?

Do I want to orient myself to the role, goal and context where I can "be" in my inter-person system, with the ability to join (or start) a subgroup?

Locating our role-system on the map will tell us where we are and "who" we are simply by observing the way we behave in our role. For example, if we are focusing on our self-development with curiosity, we are in a "developing" inner-person role that can lead to personal insight. If we have the same inner-person focus without curiosity, we are in our "closed" survivor role, safe from any personal insights. If we are in a "personalizing" role, are we trying to understand something about our own dynamics, or are we taking something "just personally" and feeling threatened or angry? The first would be an inner-person driving force towards self-development. The second would be a restraining force to self-development but a driving force in closing boundaries to threatening inputs that would otherwise destabilize our system. By observing the characteristics of our role-system behavior, we can surmise whether it will serve as a driving or a restraining force in relationship to its goals and to the goals of its larger context.

Rather than encouraging explanation of one's history as if it is the "reason" for one's problems today, SCT emphasizes seeing one's history and exploring it from the perspective of the different contexts within the developmental journey. SCT encourages exploring experience rather than explaining it. When people cross the threshold from explaining their inner-person experience to exploring it, they have taken their first step in systems-centered therapy and their "history" changes at each new insight. The challenge of opening to new insight is that one has to be able to "sit at the edge of the unknown," a process that is made easier in the co-regulating context of functional subgrouping.

A short version of our role-systems map for everyday life

We have taken one more step to put our role-systems map into everyday life to make it easier to recognize the inherent conflicts that we all have as human beings (see Figures 5.3 and 5.7). Each system contains differences related to the different goals that each system has. Seeing these differences helped us to understand the inevitable conflicts that arise in the process of the ongoing integration of the differences within and between each system level. This then contextualizes the ongoing challenges of accessing the differences in each system and role-system and using them as driving forces for overall system development. This is especially important today with the conflicts in the world that resonate with and are isomorphic to these everyday challenges of being a human being. Seeing ourselves in our different role-systems offers a way of seeing the difference in *me* and the difference of being *we*, leading us to the ongoing human challenge of integrating differences to make a difference for how our world can *be*, so that it develops and transforms *we* and *me*.

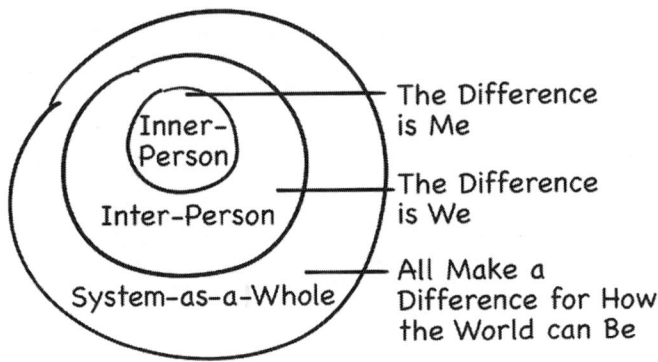

Figure 5.7

Summary

Using our illustration as a map for identifying and tracking the role–system that is active in us, in others and in our context has proven enormously valuable to us in our work. Using this map has helped us develop our inter–person observer and researcher roles. And just as important, this mapping work has led to a more in–depth exploration and understanding of the inner–person system and inner–person roles. This is the focus in our next chapter.

Working with this map lays the foundation for our work in Chapter 6 on mapping our inner–person system in greater depth and supporting our exploration of how our two different kinds of roles develop: our affiliative/attachment roles and social roles.

References

Agazarian, Y. M., & Gantt, S. P. (2014). Systems-centered training with couples: Building marriages that work. *Systemic Thinking & Psychotherapy*, *5*.

Agazarian, Y. M., & Peters, R. (1981). *The visible and invisible group*. London, UK: Routledge & Kegan Paul. Reprinted in paperback (1987). London, UK: Karnac Books.

Gantt, S. P. (2013). Applying systems-centered theory (SCT) and methods in organizational contexts: Putting SCT to work. *International Journal of Group Psychotherapy*, *63*(2), 234–258. doi:10.1521/ijgp.2013.63.2.234

Lewin, K. (1951). *Field theory in social science*. New York, NY: Harper & Row.

Porges, S. W. (1995). Orienting in a defensive world: Mammalian modifications of our evolutionary heritage: A polyvagal theory. *Psychophysiology*, *32*(4), 301–318. doi:10.1111/j.1469-8986.1995.tb01213.x

Porges, S. W. (2007). The polyvagal perspective. *Biological Psychology*, *74*(2), 116–143. doi:10.1016/j.biopsycho.2006.06.009

Porges, S. W. (2009). Stress and parasympathetic control. In L. R. Squire (Ed.), *Encyclopedia of neuroscience* (Vol. 9, pp. 463–469). Oxford, UK: Academic Press.

Porges, S. W. (2011). *The polyvagal theory: Neurophysiological foundations of emotions, attachment, communication, and self-regulation*. New York, NY: Norton.

Shannon, C. E., & Weaver, W. (1964). *The mathematical theory of communication*. Urbana, IL: University of Illinois Press.

Simon, A., & Agazarian, Y. M. (1967). *SAVI: Sequential analysis of verbal interaction*. Philadelphia, PA: Research for Better Schools.

Chapter 6

Exploring our inner-person system roles

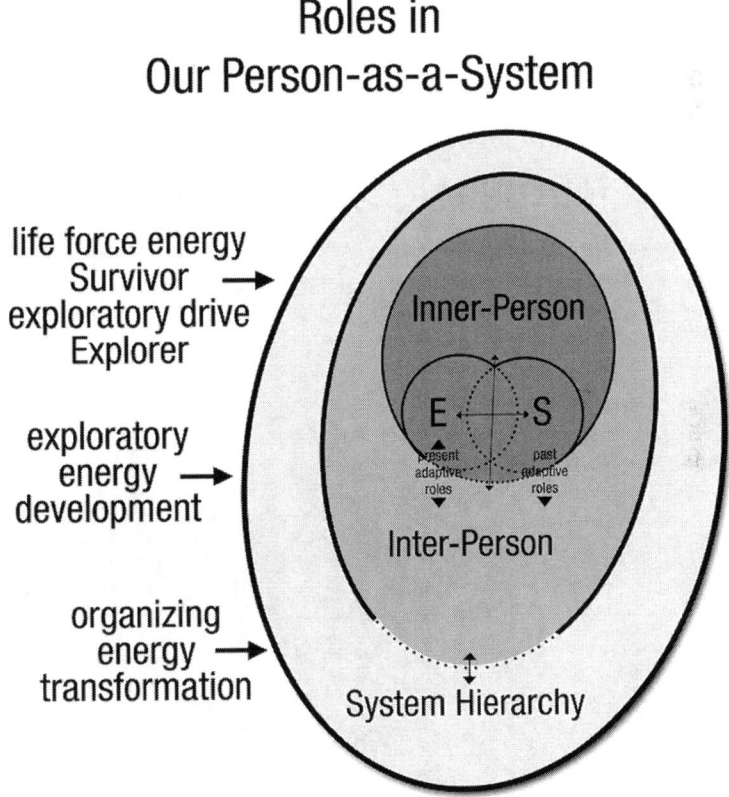

Roles in Our Person-as-a-System

life force energy
Survivor ⟶
exploratory drive
Explorer

exploratory
energy ⟶
development

organizing
energy ⟶
transformation

Inner-Person

E ⟵ ⟶ S

present
adaptive
roles

past
adaptive
roles

Inter-Person

System Hierarchy

Figure 6.1

Past adaptive roles, as we noted in Chapter 4, originally develop in the inner-person survivor system under two different conditions: threat and no threat. When the survivor system is secure and without threat, we are in our primary person survivor roles, where our boundaries can open and close and are potentially permeable to the exploratory drive as well as the life force energy (see Figure 6.1). In contrast, our past adaptive roles which we also call secondary survivor roles have mostly closed boundaries (open only to confirming similarities) with little or no access to the exploratory drive. Our survivor roles include two kinds of role-systems: our affiliative/attachment roles and our social roles.

Our two kinds of survivor roles: affiliative/ attachment and social

Our two kinds of survivor roles organize our different energies. Affiliative/ attachment roles relate primarily to the life force. Social roles relate to both the life force and the exploratory drive. Affiliative/attachment roles develop first within the self-centered system in the survivor system. Social roles develop later as the child grows older, with boundaries potentially permeable to both the inner life force and the exploratory drive, fueling interactions with others. These social roles develop at the boundary between the inner- and inter-person (see Figure 6.2).

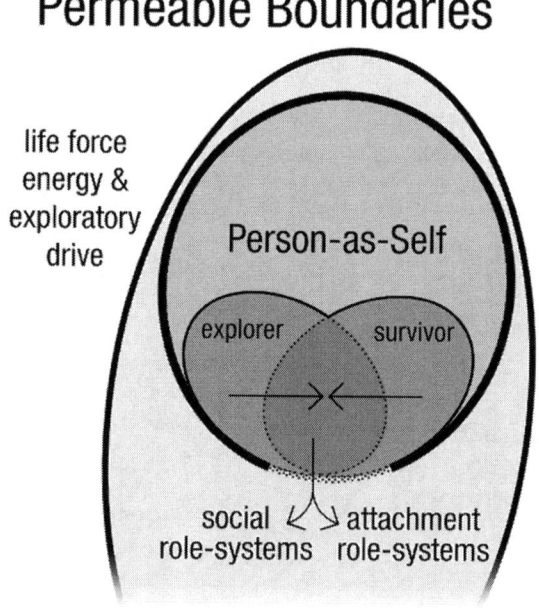

Figure 6.2

These two different kinds of roles are similar in that both kinds of roles develop and activate under threat and conflict. Yet these role-systems develop differently in that they develop in two different conflictual contexts: when conflicts arise from failures in resonant affiliation or from conflicts between attunement and socialization goals.

Developing first, our affiliative/attachment role-systems are our earliest role-systems. These develop when there is a failure in resonance that is not repaired and the personalized self (closed boundaries) preempts the functioning of our primary affiliation self (where boundaries can open and close).

Social roles relate to conflicts that occur when the child is confronted by the socializing demands with their significant parenting figures, a marked difference from reliable attunement without requirements. In this context, social role-systems with closed boundaries develop when empathy fails and resonance and attunement become contingent on compliance. Social roles are developmentally later, when the socialization goals have become important.

As we have emphasized, maintaining equilibrium is basic to survival; thus, closing boundaries to all destabilizing inputs is a driving force for survival. First and foremost is the reality that repeating roles from the past is a repetition compulsion that originally allowed us to compromise between maintaining enough affiliative connection with our significant others and at the same time responding to the contingent demands of a relationship with someone separate from us.

In both sets of conflicts, the difference from outside ourselves is too different from "us," and this difference is then experienced as a threat, leading to closed boundaried survivor role-systems! We developed these secondary survivor role-systems in our childhood to defend and protect ourselves from these early traumas around loss of resonance. These role-systems are with us today and have been the foundation upon which many of our roles have been built.

The sad fact is that, though adaptive in the past, these secondary roles are rarely adaptive in the present. Instead, in the present, they are the roles of the repetition compulsion and often serve as role inductions to others into "old" survivor roles that repeat the past in the present at the cost of development.

Moving beyond scapegoating our own defenses: seeing the system context of our role-systems

Though the differences that trigger our secondary survivor role-systems are typically differences from outside of us, we also get triggered by internal differences. Our role-system response then is even more of a challenge as the differences within oneself are held in a subsystem role in our inner-person behind closed boundaries and scapegoated (see Figure 6.3).

For example, these encapsulations happen when we disapprove of our own anger and fail to recognize our anger as the energy of the life force, feel guilty about our thoughts and miss seeing them as a signal for testing reality, or ward off an event with disassociating shame instead of staying curious. When we frame these early adaptive role-systems as "defenses," we are already reacting to them and scapegoating them, just as we described doing in our large group in Chapter 3.

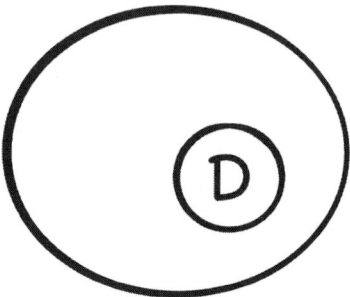

Figure 6.3

Introducing the idea of role-systems and learning to map them is making it easier to explore our knee-jerk reactions to our human experiences. We can then activate more of our curiosity instead of just reactivity. What is more, by introducing roles as systems we have also introduced the potential for viewing them as driving and/or restraining forces, not only in relationship to the goals of the role itself but also, thanks to Lewin (1951), in relationship to the goals of our inner-person, inter-person or whole person of which our role-systems are an output. In short, by "seeing" role-systems, we are moving away from enacting our survivor roles of scapegoating ourselves and into a curious explorer role. It was only after we understood more about the fundamental differences in the role-systems that develop from conflicts in empathic attunement and in the inter-person demands of socializing that we came to realize that survivor system boundaries are only permeable to the life force communications of empathic attunement. Even empathic words can fail to reach us when we experience ourselves fighting for our lives.

Bringing our role-systems map to life: how our inner-person role-systems develop

Using our role-systems map (see Figure 6.4) has furthered our focus on the development of our early role-systems. To reiterate, all secondary survivor roles, past or present, were originally adaptive compromises for containing conflict between two competing and conflicting goals, both of which are important to the system survival. Roles imported from the past have boundaries that are selectively permeable, open to inputs from the context that are similar enough to the original role organization and closed to the differences which could potentially lead to change. All roles were once a solution, however maladaptive they are in the present. Early roles are useful compromises developed to respond to the role requirements of an important relationship.

Our earliest conflicts relate to maintaining the symbiotic equilibrium in our inner-person while relating to our necessary parenting others. Resonance and attunement always fluctuate in the symbiotic system of "child and parent." Both

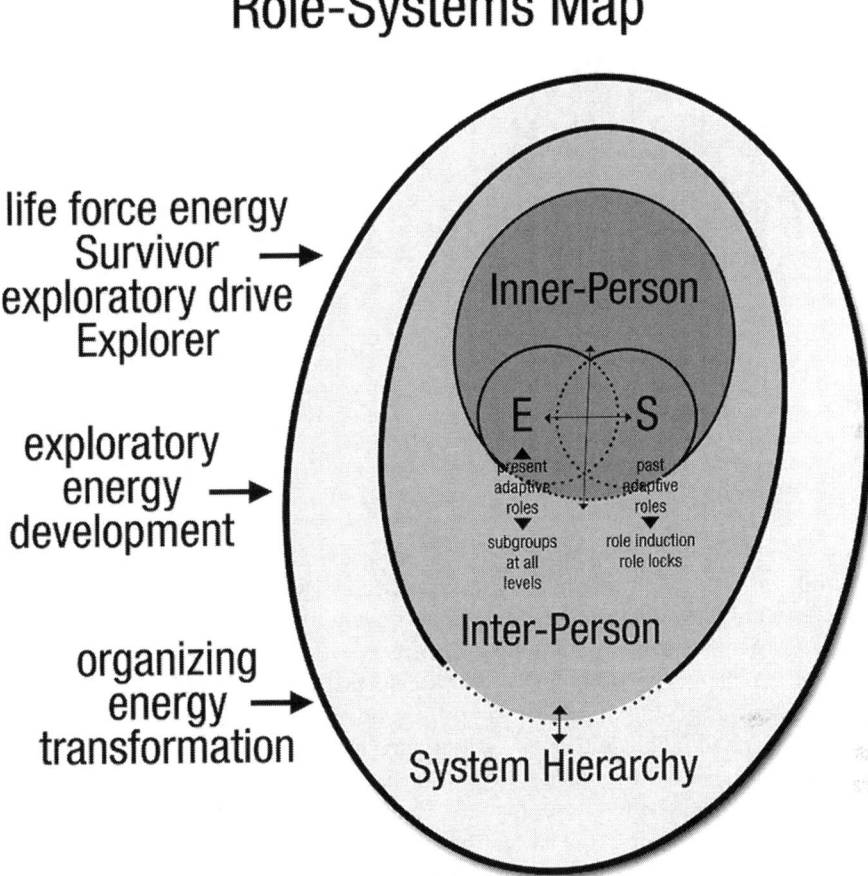

Role-Systems Map

life force energy
Survivor →
exploratory drive
Explorer

exploratory
energy →
development

organizing
energy →
transformation

Inner-Person

E ←→ S

present
adaptive
roles

past
adaptive
roles

subgroups
at all
levels

role induction
role locks

Inter-Person

System Hierarchy

Figure 6.4

the child/parent system and also the nascent system of the child must titrate these fluctuations. This is the context in which our inner-person primary and secondary affiliative/attachment role-systems develop (see Figure 6.5). For those parenting people who are open to their own care-giving system in their inner-person roles, the early symbiotic system of "child and parent" is an easier time as the resonance and attunement to the child and her or his care-seeking comes easily for this subgroup. The same subgroup is often more challenged when the goals shift to socializing, where attunement from the parent becomes contingent on the child cooperating. (This is one of the places where having a parenting system with two different roles with differential resources can be so helpful: often one parent has more accessibility to care-giving and the other more of the needed "resolve" for socialization.)

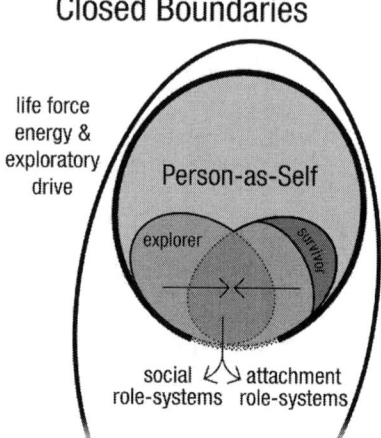

Permeable Boundaries

life force
energy &
exploratory
drive

Person-as-Self

explorer   survivor

social ⤵⤴ attachment
role-systems   role-systems

Closed Boundaries

life force
energy &
exploratory
drive

Person-as-Self

explorer   survivor

social ⤵⤴ attachment
role-systems   role-systems

Figure 6.5

In the socialization context, the parenting goals expand to include socializing the child, as when, for example, the young child system is taught not to bite. As biting is natural behavior and self-expression in the developmental process for all baby animals, socializing a child away from biting can be experienced as a violation of the innate expression of the inner-person self. This example well illustrates the inevitable conflict between our impulses and the requirement that we control them. We are all taught in our early years not to bite others, in spite of the fact that biting is a natural stage of development in all young animals (anyone who has had a puppy or kitten remembers this!). Our social roles are always compromise solutions to the conflict between our "want" for unconditional positive regard and care-giving and the demands from our significant others that we develop socially.

Our inner-person experiences the disruption of the socializing demands and, if all goes well enough, we learn to cooperate from our developing inter-person. When our essential self *is* violated, the difference is too great and there is a threatening conflict between the affiliation system and the social system. It is in this threatening conflict that secondary survivor roles develop in order to maintain the two essential connections. Whether this is traumatic depends upon whether the socializing roles contain shame or whether, after the social input, there is repair in the relational system. For example, a mother was socializing her son to eat his lunch when he only wanted to eat chips. The mother made chips contingent on eating half a sandwich. The child complied (a role) and then glared intently at the mother. The mother told him why she required him to eat: so that he would not get tired later. She then hugged the child; he responded affectionately, shifting from his angry glare to smiling at the restoration of the affiliative relationship which had been temporarily ruptured when the socialization took priority. In the repair, the differences in the affiliative and socialization goals were integrated (Gantt, in press).

First role-systems: affiliative/attachment

We have conceptualized affiliative/attachment role-systems in our inner-person survivor system as fueled by our life force energy (see Figure 6.6). Our name for these role-systems reflects how our theorizing has drawn upon the research in the attachment field and translated it into systems language to deepen our thinking about these role-systems.

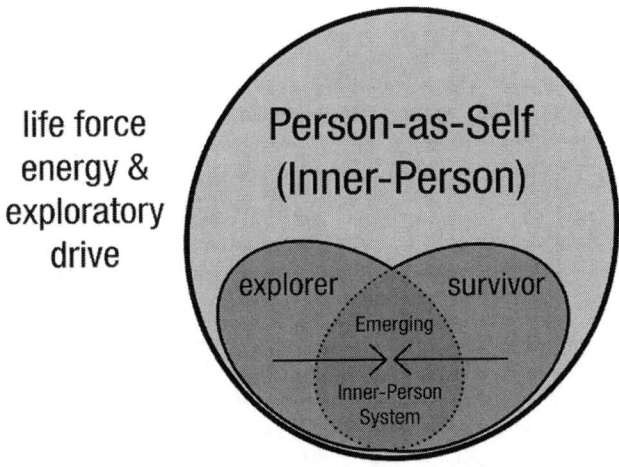

life force
energy &
exploratory
drive

Person-as-Self
(Inner-Person)

explorer   survivor

Emerging

Inner-Person
System

Figure 6.6

Care-giving and care-seeking as primary survivor roles

Though our work of conceptualizing affiliative/attachment *role-systems* is unique to SCT, not surprisingly, as the name "affiliative/attachment" suggests, we have been influenced by the attachment literature pioneered by Bowlby (1969, 1979, 1982, 1988). This literature describes how, under threat, our care-seeking activates and we seek protection and care, whether in situations which threaten life or under conditions of extreme fatigue or fear or separation or ordinary anxiety or even, as we know from interpersonal neurobiology, in regulating our feelings. Early in our life, our survival necessitates mothering/fathering containment and regulation of our feelings as our baby brain is not yet developed. As both our baby brain and our adult brain are social brains (Cozolino, 2010, 2012, 2014), co-regulating is our birthright. This early co-regulating is the inter-person context in which the inner-person survivor roles develop. These earliest roles include neuronal firing patterns which provide a role-system template for subsequent roles as we internalize the co-regulating that we experience and learn with our parenting figures (Badenoch, 2017). Again, drawing from interpersonal neurobiology, our parenting figures' brains regulate ours in a right brain to right brain pattern of implicit regulation (Schore, 2019a). This regulating process shapes our brain and is the context in which our primary and secondary survivor roles first develop. This co-regulating, which is inter-person system regulation (right to right brain), is vital for the inner-person system survival and development. In addition, this is nicely compatible with Porges' (2007, 2011) work on our nervous system preference to regulate in connection with others rather than relying only on our other autonomic nervous system potentials like flight, fight or freeze.

Seeing care-seeking and care-giving through a systems-centered lens

Care-seeking and care-giving are two sides of the same attachment coin or, translated to systems theory, two functional roles that support our attachment goals which relate to both survival and development. Each role has its own goal which is to give care or to receive care, respectively. It is of immense significance that these role-systems remain "turned on" until they reach their goal. Reaching the goal requires inter-person cooperation. If the goal is *not* met, this dynamic will fuel or activate the secondary (more closed) survivor role-systems like identified patient and helper. We are reminded here of Lewin's (1951) tension system between the goal and the person that is satisfied only when the person reaches the goal. We have been helped in our understanding of these dynamics by not only Bowlby (1969, 1979, 1982, 1988) but also the work of Dorothy Heard and Brian Lake (1986, 1997) and Una McCluskey (2002, 2005). These influences have led us to focus on care-giving and care-seeking as the primary attachment dynamics that relate to the development of our affiliative/attachment role-systems. Affiliative/attachment role-systems with their goal of survival enable us to get protection and emotional regulation, both in the inner-person (child) and inter-person (mother–child system) systems.

It is in our nascent survivor system that the role-systems of affiliation/attachment develop in the symbiotic connection with the mother or other primary care-givers (right to right brain). This early symbiotic system enables our autonomic nervous system and limbic system and resonance circuitry to develop, which makes it possible to have resonant and attuned role-systems with ourselves and others. Later in our development, as our prefrontal cortex matures, we also develop our ability to experience empathic role-systems. Our affiliative/attachment roles develop in an interactive context[1] in our survivor self or role-system, fueled by the life force, rooted in the empathic attunement that begins before we are born. They are the source of our security and our ability to relate to ourselves and others.

Even more important, when activated, the care-seeking, care-giving systems fueled by the life force take precedence over the exploratory drive. To oversimplify, building on the attachment literature, we would say that when the goal-directed care-seeking, care-giving roles are turned on, the exploratory drive is turned off. The success of all SCT methods is dependent upon the activation of curiosity from the centered system as an alternative to becoming imprisoned in maladaptive roles. So, it is of great significance in SCT that the arousal of care-seeking and care-giving roles in one's survivor system trigger the deactivation of the necessary curiosity that accompanies the exploratory drive if it is not satisfied. Without security, we are not exploratory, and our survivor roles have only the goal of surviving!

Functional subgrouping: lowering threat and building a secure context

This is where the significance of functional subgrouping is so important in that subgrouping functionally changes the context towards one of greater resonance and hence greater security. By initiating functional subgrouping from the beginning of all groups and each session of group, fear responses are less likely to be aroused or more easily lowered when arousal does occur. Theoretically, functional subgrouping lowers entropic noise (ambiguity, contradiction, redundancy). We have also suggested earlier that the subgroup makes a secure enough environment that the exploratory drive activates (Gantt & Agazarian, 2010, 2011). In our newer theory, we can also articulate that functional subgrouping develops a functional inter-person role-system. This inter-person role is a containing and developing context for the inner-person and potentiates greater attunement and resonance, making it more possible to become curious and relate from a primary survivor role and a curious explorer role, fueling and fueled by the developing inter-person system.

The development of different social roles (inter-person) is essential for development at all system levels. Functional subgrouping roles are SCT's primary social roles! Functional subgrouping makes it more possible to integrate the differences in the conflicts that our secondary survivor role-systems originally managed. At the same time, functional subgrouping develops our social brain resources and our capacity for co-regulating (Gantt, 2019a; Gantt & Badenoch, 2020).

When we reflect the other person in the functional subgrouping process, the goal of the interactive system is for the "talker" to be understood, however much back-and-forth this takes. This reflection process starts to build a "secure base" (Gantt, 2018) by developing the "secure inter-person system." Functional subgrouping provides a secure base which contains the inner-person system with its primary and secondary affiliative/attachment role-systems. This more secure subgroup system then makes it possible for the boundary in the secondary roles to become more permeable to our explorer system and its curiosity, so essential for our development. Our attachment roles are stimulated by context – when the context is one in which we are in empathic attunement with others "all is well" (primary rather than secondary roles depending upon role-system capacity). In our primary attachment roles with others, our exploratory drive increases and our fear responses go down, and our survivor role-system can integrate small differences and develop.

The right hemisphere and functional subgrouping

Our deepening understanding of the right hemisphere has increased our appreciation of the impact of functional subgrouping and its potential for developing our survivor roles. We have emphasized in earlier work the importance of the right hemisphere for implicit learning and emotional co-regulation (Gantt, 2018; Gantt & Badenoch, 2020) and the centrality of our implicit right brain function for our well-being and co-regulation with others. It is useful here to briefly summarize in more depth how our hemispheres function differently, that is, how each hemisphere plays a different role.

Our two different hemispheres see and function differently

McGilchrist's (2009) groundbreaking work has highlighted the different ways of attending, then perceiving, and thus experiencing in our two hemispheres. Thinking systems, we can conceptualize each hemisphere as a different subsystem and different context with different perceptions and experience inside the person system. The right hemisphere orients to relational space and when responded to by others in attunement, we are regulated. The autonomic ventral vagal circuits active in social engagement (Porges, 2007, 2011) are more right-centric, just as is our knowing by sensing or getting a feel of something (in SCT, we call this apprehending). As Badenoch (2017) describes it:

> These two different ways of attending are supported by the multiple connections between the cortical columns in the right hemisphere and the relatively isolated columns in the left (Hawkins & Blakeslee, 2004; McGilchrist, 2009). Most simply, we can say that the right hemisphere contains significantly more white matter because the cortical columns of neurons are richly interconnected. These pathways are then myelinated, both increasing synaptic strength and speeding movement throughout these well-wired networks. In this way, experience coming in or being recalled is held in the larger neuronal context and may be felt more as spreading waves in the body than as isolated particles of information (to borrow a metaphor from quantum physics). On the left, these columns are much more like silos with far fewer interconnections. This serves well to order information in a way that allows us to take bits and pieces and rearrange them into new fixed patterns to achieve the goal we have identified. Additionally, new information coming in from the senses has a tendency to be perceived as bits of information rather than a flowing stream, with these bits getting sorted according to the categories already encoded in these silos. . . . . Difficulties arise when the *relationship* between the hemispheres is altered in ways that prevent them from having an ongoing conversation that supports collaborative expression of their unique gifts.
>
> (pp. 6–7)

Returning to what we introduced in Chapter 4, Schore, in his seminal work, has reconceptualized the unconscious as a relational unconscious where we communicate right brain to right brain. This right-to-right brain communication happens initially in our earliest attachment relationship where "communicating brains align and synchronize their neural activities with other brains" (2019a, p. 15). Right brain function dominates in babies as the left brain function is slower to develop and the infant relies on the mothering figure for right-to-right regulating. This right-to-right regulation establishes our early attachment patterns, yet our relational unconscious communication (right-to-right) continues throughout our life span. For example, Schore (2019a, 2019b) sees this synchrony between right brains as central in the therapeutic process where right-to-right communication functions as a regulatory process and simultaneously supports implicit right brain development. He also has focused his work on the "synchronized, right-lateralized interbrain communication of emotions within the co-constructed attachment relationship embedded in the therapeutic alliance" (2019a, p. 11). Similarly, Badenoch (2011, 2017), in her discussion of the primacy of co-regulation, describes how in our optimal functioning, we are always co-regulating either with the internalized other when we are alone or in the moment-to-moment flow between us and others.

In contrast, our left brain is highly resourceful in organizing systems and algorithms and generalizations from data and in problem-solving by putting pieces together. McGilchrist (2009) has articulated many ways in which our culture is now left brain–dominated and impacting us all the time, influencing us to split off from feeling connected with others and instead becoming more wary.

Functional subgrouping develops the right hemisphere

In SCT, we have linked these important understandings to the process of functional subgrouping which, from this framework, can be seen as providing a practicum in right-to-right brain co-regulation. Functional subgrouping not only increases the likelihood of verbal communication but also functions as a neural exercise that is strengthening right-to-right brain implicit communication, nonverbal communication and our capacity for resonance and attunement with ourselves and others (Gantt, 2019b). This is exciting to us, as it starts to put a comprehension (left brain) around what we have long apprehended (right brain). In fact, we would say that functional subgrouping provides practice in interpersonal synchronizations that Schore (2019a) has stressed are vital in emotional communications. These understandings of the centrality of right brain communication have laid a vital foundation for deepening our work with affiliative/attachment roles.

Primary and secondary affiliative/attachment roles

Affiliation/attachment role-systems relate to the goal of survival through satisfying our care-giving/care-seeking or at least making the best satisfaction possible in our interactive mother–child system. Drawing again from Schore's work, these roles are essential as they relate to our adaptations beginning when "the mother shapes limbic-autonomic circuits in the infant's early developing right hemisphere" (2019a, p. 1). Affiliative/attachment role-systems develop from our beginnings *and* contain us to change throughout life. As in all role-systems that develop as adaptations to our past contexts, nascent affiliative/attachment responses are the precursor to *all* later role-systems. Affiliation/attachment role-systems speak an unspoken language. All affiliative/attachment role-systems "know" without words and are fueled by the apprehensive knowing of our life force. In our primary affiliative/attachment roles, we seek care and give care in resonance with others. In our secondary or closed roles, we live in survival through our past adaptations.

Primary affiliative/attachment roles

Our primary role-systems have boundaries that are responsive to the life force, opening and closing, as relevant to our context, to our life force energy and exploratory drive. These primary roles are the source of our security and our ability to relate to ourselves and others. They contain both our care-giving and care-seeking roles fueled by the life force. Our primary attachment roles are available to us whenever we are in empathic attunement with others and are "triggered" so to speak, whenever there is good enough attunement. It is by remaining connected to the life force within these roles that we develop our true self. Without these roles, we would not have survived, as our human species is dependent on care from others and these roles maintain the caring system (care-giving and care-taking roles) and its vital relationships. This circles us back again to the potency of functional subgrouping as it can restore our empathic attunement with others that is our birthright. In addition, functional subgrouping trains our inborn capacity for co-regulating. This weakens the pull to our secondary affiliative/attachment roles as the co-regulation in sub-grouping provides an alternative to our secondary survivor roles and is a here-and-now adaptation which develops our primary roles.

Though SCT first works explicitly in therapy and consultation with the restraining forces in social roles and simultaneously develops SCT's social role of functional subgrouping, our attachment role-systems actually develop first, at the beginning of our life, and are likely even primed in utero. Stress (in utero as well as after birth) can influence the exploratory drive and/or fear linked to our survivor roles. For example, we can be born with high exploration and low fear or vice versa. As an infant, we then develop in relationship to our context, seeking care from our care-giver(s).

Our secondary affiliative/attachment roles

Typical of past adaptive role-systems, our secondary affiliative/attachment survivor role-systems come and go, aroused under stress, by conflicting differences, by separation or threat, or by the phase of a group or a couple or even the therapeutic system. When we are in these past adaptations, our boundaries are only open to information that confirms our secondary role and closed to any differences that might disconfirm it, a selective boundary permeability so to speak. In the past, this selective permeability developed in the service of system stability and survival.

As Porges described in his foreword to Badenoch's book (2017):

> ... the emergent properties of defensive states functionally transform the individual from a social being into a solitary individual. Defensive strategies encapsulate the individual and limit options for neurophysiological regulation from co-regulation to a more inefficient and limited mode of self-regulation. ... Although this shift in neural state optimizes survival through defensive strategies, survival needs of co-regulation and connectedness are compromised. As defense is optimized, it reflexively dominates personal experience and limits the neural resources that foster social interactions and co-regulation.
>
> (pp. x–xi)

In many ways, Porges' descriptive of defensive states is an excellent operational definition of our secondary survivor roles. Importantly, our systems perspective adds an essential difference as well: we reframe these patterns as *role-systems*, with identifiable behaviors, attitudes, cognitive capacity and inner experience that can be linked to an identifiable trigger, usually outside oneself and very often from the phase of the context itself and its phase dynamics. What is also vital is that our systems perspective reframes "defensive states" in systems language as closed survivor roles that were driving forces when initially developed and are now restraining to present problem-solving. This systems view is normalizing, making it easier to be curious about our roles instead of defensive. What is similar to Porges is that SCT emphasizes co-regulation as fundamental to all living human systems.

Working with affiliative/attachment roles

Whereas with social roles, readiness for change is assessed in terms of the developmental phase, the deeper roots of our secondary affiliative/attachment roles are not addressed until there is an attuned and empathic connection established in the therapeutic system. Also, SCT does not explicitly work with exploring or weakening the restraining forces to attachment, which are rooted in the life force and our survival, until the intimacy phase of system development. By the time the system has developed to this phase, the social defenses and the defenses against authentic experience have already been modified.

The developmental work in the intimacy phase is the exploration of separation and individuation issues and our human conflicts around wanting to be close or distant, easily enacted in a role lock with one person moving towards to be closer and the other pushing away (see Figure 6.7).

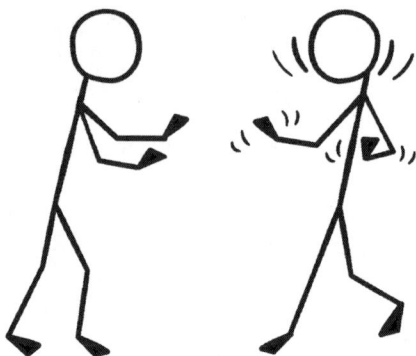

Figure 6.7

These conflicts are implicit in our affiliative/attachment roles that developed as our role adaptations to ruptures in care-giving/care-seeking system, for example, always managing alone and never being alone.

Usefully in SCT, these conflicts and our early role adaptations often emerge in the steps of functional subgrouping (Gantt, in press). The work with the functional subgrouping protocol in the earlier phases of group is learning to subgroup. In the intimacy phase, the protocol can then be used as a diagnostic tool for identifying the role-systems that are triggered in the steps of the protocol which require a series of separations and individuations in the process of co-regulating. Functional subgroups then form to explore the challenges and the secondary adaptations that arise when observing the roles that are aroused at each step in the subgrouping protocol.

Using functional subgrouping and the person-as-a-system map to explore affiliative/attachment roles

Seeing the functional subgrouping protocol from the person-as-a-system map is also useful here. The map has helped us to contextualize our human challenges in changing role-systems. Seeing where we are on the map and where we want to go has been useful in de-pathologizing the inevitable turbulence of crossing a boundary from one role-system to another. For example, in subgrouping, after a person speaks and then says "anyone else?", the person is shifting from inner-person crossing the boundary into the unknown of the inter-person context. Any silence or delay in the group's responding easily triggers a secondary past survivor role related to the challenges of being oneself with others. Or when someone is reflected and feels understood, the challenge of separating and connecting with oneself can also stimulate a secondary survivor role. Affiliative/attachment roles often emerge at each step of the protocol.

The basic steps in functional subgrouping linked to our role-systems map are:

Say "anyone else?" when you have finished saying what you want to say.
Look around so that everyone in the group feels invited to join you. [inner- to inter-person to whole system]
Don't give up if it takes time for someone to join you. [inner- to inter-person]
When you are joined, expect the person who joins you to reflect what you said.
If you don't feel joined, say so! [inner-person]
When you join someone else, reflect what they said. [inter-person]
Once you have joined [inter], separate, connect to yourself [inner] and add your similarity to the group. [inter-person and whole system]

To elaborate, the first step in subgrouping is making eye contact with the person who has spoken and reflecting the heart of his or her message. Interestingly, a recent study shows that talking face-to-face predicts greater brain synchrony (Dikker et al., 2017). Making eye contact is an inter-person activity, yet it requires centering into our curious explorer to empathically attune, empathize and open to the other's life force. Without our explorer, our paraphrase will be pro forma, letter of the law, and without the heart of the message or, as our axiom says, words without feelings have no meaning. The heart of reflecting is synchronizing, both words but most importantly the implicit right-to-right brain resonance and attunement.

Subgroups can form to explore what happens for each member in reflecting. Some members shift into observing (inter-person role) and explore their secondary affiliative/attachment survivor role that is triggered when the task is to reflect the other and the other's feelings. For example, members discover the pull to stay with themselves and keep their boundary closed to the other, while others easily paraphrase the other's words but stay closed to the other's feelings. Some members start to notice keeping out similarities, a survivor role with the goal of staying safe by staying different. All of these are outputs from secondary affiliative/attachment role-systems.

The next step in subgrouping is separating after a successful reflection, which requires shifting from the connection with the other to a centering connection with oneself. Separating from the other can be challenging, as it is hard to move away from a well-earned connection and in many early survivor roles, the adaptation was to avoid separating. Centering into connection with oneself is another common context where our secondary affiliative/attachment roles may emerge as there is often a subgroup who adapted by not connecting to themselves and only orienting to others' feelings.

Adding something from one's centered self-connection that builds on the similarity while adding small differences is also an important step towards developing oneself. Adding one's build into the group and staying curiously open in the unknown to see how the group responds can also arouse our secondary role-systems that we developed in our early life around separation and individuation.

Seeing our affiliative/attachment roles and their implications in context

As we have discussed previously, every role can serve as a driving or a restraining force depending upon the goals of the context. When all goes well, our roles reflect responses that are congruent with the goals of our transforming, centered system, enabling satisfying care-giving and care-seeking interactions that then support an openness to our exploratory drive. When the goal is to maintain the system status quo, threatened by differences too great to integrate, secondary attachment roles serve as a driving force. When on the other hand the goal is not only survival but also development, the goal is better served by opening boundaries to curiosity about the context of the threat. In this case, the closed secondary roles are a fixating restraining force. Without curiosity about either ourselves or others, we tend to make "as if" relationships. In groups, we develop "as if" subgroups.

In SCT, we do not think about role behaviors as symptoms of pathology. We think about them as common, normal, universal behaviors that signal who we are at any one particular time and also tell us about the goals of the system that sponsors them. Even more important, they signal the developmental dynamics and they let us know whether we are responding with past or present roles.

When all does not go well, our secondary affiliative/attachment roles fuel and become part of a dominant-submissive social role relationship and lead to role locks. For example, when our care-seeking is aroused and the response is words without feeling, our care-seeking is frustrated. Or if our care-giving is aroused and all offers of care are rebuked, our care-giving is frustrated. In both, the care-giving and care-seeking impulses have no satisfactory outlet, resulting in the goals remaining frustrated with survivor roles activated. All of this is at the expense of the exploratory drive. When our closed survivor role-systems are mobilized, the care-seeking energy can then be obscured in a past adaptive helpless role and its reciprocal role, the care-giving system, in a past adaptive helping or care-taking role, often leading to a role lock.

More learning from our training groups

Our training groups have once again been invaluable in these explorations. As they discovered, when we are confronted with misattunements (which is always a difference), we easily "feel" as if the misattunement is a threat to our survival. In real life, we take things that threaten us very personally and close our minds (an effective way of closing our system boundaries) to anything that does not fit us. Yet no human is an island. Personalizing (closing our boundary) works in the short run, but not in the long run, because when we personalize, we have no curiosity. We need curiosity to develop ourselves and our role-systems. To have curiosity available requires, as the attachment literature describes it, a "secure base." We need our curiosity if we are to observe and to develop not only ourselves but also our social relationships with the outside world. Our curious explorer self can open our boundaries to being socialized. This is where functional subgrouping has made it possible for us to work in a different way with role-systems as functional subgrouping provides a secure inter-person base that contains and develops the inner-person roles. This supports exploration and, at the same time, exploring our role responses in each step of subgrouping gives us a useful way to explore our affiliative/attachment role-systems in the here-and-now.

De-pathologizing our affiliation reactions

We cannot help that our human species takes things just personally and we retreat into our inner-person self-centered system when our emotional interactions violate our expectations and our feelings get hurt. This has been vital in our past to our survival, yet what is much more important is to survive and develop rather than personalizing something about ourselves or the other who disappointed us.

Linking back to our theory has been helpful in understanding the prototypic triggers for our affiliative/attachment roles. Not surprisingly, noise (ambiguity, contradiction, redundancy) in the communication channel will trigger our past adaptive closed affiliate/attachment roles. Noise is a role-system output from a closed survivor role so that the induction to the receiving system often triggers a reciprocal closed survivor role. For example, our closed attachment roles are triggered "when the words don't match the music or emotion" (contradiction), when the other's face is blank (ambiguity), or when there are many words yet no feelings (redundancy).

Our newer perspective on role-systems is proving useful in systems-centered practice, whether it is for training or therapy or personal growth or even in diagnosing an organizational team's capacity to change. For example, when our feelings get hurt and we take everything personally, if we can become curious, we can shift to observing ourselves relating in our inner-person system from our survival subsystem. As we are observing, we are shifting into our inter-person system where we can collect data rather than closing our boundary. With our curiosity available, we can think about the possibility that we are experiencing our survival as if it is under threat. By becoming curious about our reactions, we have shifted from subjective experience (inner-person) which often has no words, to include objective experience (inter-person) which allows us to think and assess the reality. We can then wonder what the stimulus was for our personal or impersonal reaction. Was the stimulus a "look-alike" in the present that repeated an inter-personal conflict from the past, or was it a present role induction from another's past role? Objectifying our role responses is a different experience from our "hurt feelings" reactions. We have also changed the potential for resolving the transfer of outputs and inputs from one system to another and altering the impact of the role induction.

Social role-systems

Though affiliative/attachment roles develop in early life before the social roles, in SCT practice, we actually focus our early work on socializing dynamics and social roles. We modify the restraining forces of the secondary social role-systems immediately from the beginning of therapy before working with the attachment role-systems that relate more deeply to the inner experience of the person. By focusing on socializing dynamics first before the attachment issues, we are working in the present with the defenses that are the easiest to weaken. Working with the social roles develops the inter-person system, which builds a containing and developing context for the later work with inner-person roles. Thus, the work on recognizing and undoing social roles builds the resources for subsequent work on the affiliation issues that relate more deeply to the inner experience of the person.

Thinking in terms of our role-systems map (refer again to Figure 6.4), the roles in each system level will be isomorphic with each other, that is, similar in

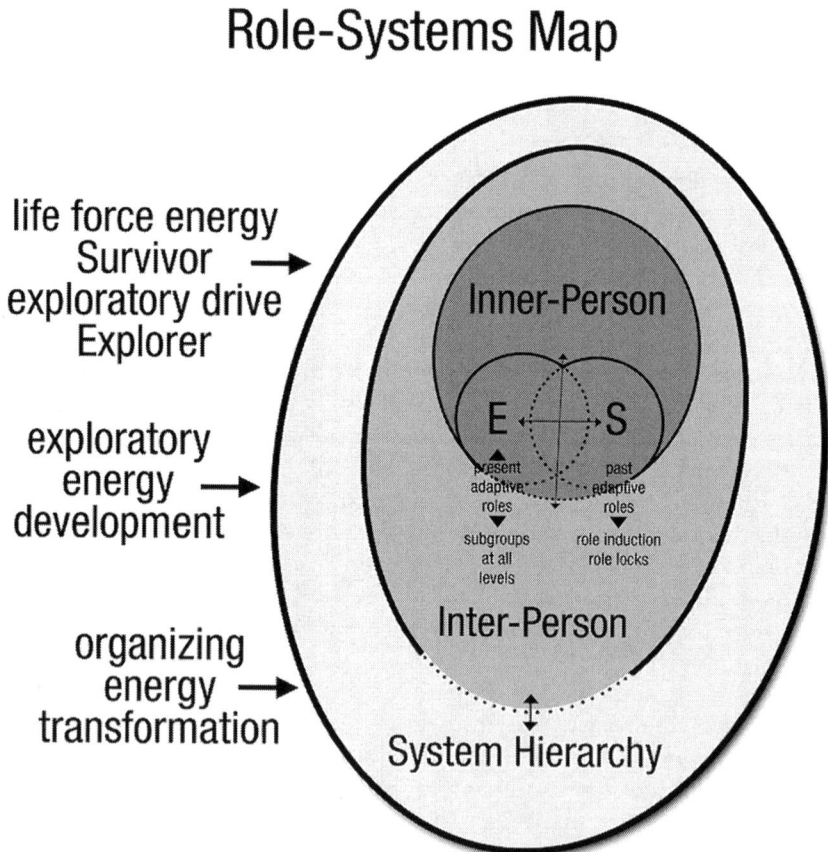

Figure 6.4

structure and function and different in different contexts, including the context of the phase of development. For example, there is isomorphy between our affiliative/attachment roles and our social roles in our inner-person and inter-person systems, respectively. Also, importantly, our social roles tend to emerge early in the sequence of the phases of system development and at the same time, there will be isomorphy between our social roles in the authority phase and our affiliative/attachment roles in the intimacy phase.

In organizations, the work with social roles is the central and fundamental work. This focus is critically important, as it is past social roles that prevent us from working in the "role, goal and context" that is so essential to functioning in teams and organizations. The work with social roles is done in the context of weakening restraining forces to taking one's work role to support the goal of the context.

Social roles at the boundary of inner- and inter-person

Our social roles develop at the boundary between our inner- and inter-person and are imported into our inter-personal system. These secondary roles developed in our early past as a compromise solution to the conflict between our attachment goals and our inner sense of our own integrity and our socialization goals and the demands to conform socially. This is a challenging conflict, as it is vital for all of us to maintain the integrity of our essential self, including our "want" for unconditional positive regard and connection – this *is* our life force energy. At the same time, the people with whom we need connection are also those requiring us to modify our impulses so that we can be socialized. Our open social roles are fueled by the energy of our exploratory drive. Our closed social roles link to early compromises that were highly adaptive when they were first developed but are rarely useful in the present. Real threats and challenges in the present need present solutions. As we have emphasized, when we are in our past adaptive or secondary social roles, our resources are related to past problems, not present ones.

Secondary social roles develop when the nascent system closes its boundaries to differences that cannot be integrated (see Figure 6.8). In this case, survival comes at the price of further development as these roles then have closed boundaries. When the goal is to maintain the system status quo, threatened by differences too great to integrate, secondary social roles serve as a driving force. When, on the other hand, survival is better served by opening boundaries to curiosity about the context of the threatening difference, then these secondary social roles are a fixating restraining force.

For example, a small child may be reaching for some forbidden thing and get told "no." A typical response is for the child to drop his head in frustration with a momentary depression at his energy being blocked. If the tone of voice and the subsequent interactions are harsh or shaming, the child is likely to develop a role to contain the shame and even the depressive solution. If, on the other hand, the "no" is supportive in tone, and perhaps coupled with an approving

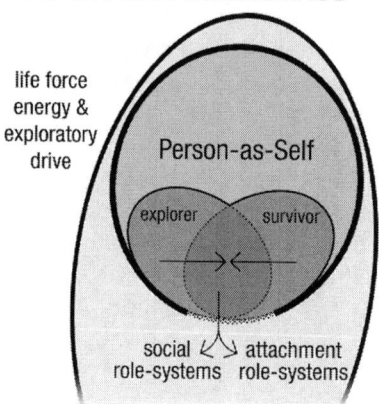

Figure 6.8

"good" when the child cooperates, the adult contributes to a system repair. With the repair, the child is not so threatened by the interaction that he has to develop a compromise role to contain the shaming. When socializing can be done in attunement to both the life force and exploratory drive, the child does not have to develop a social compliant or defiant role, and the exploratory drive is not compromised. For example, we watched in great admiration as a five-year-old lying on top of his mother would laugh and say, "tell me what I am not supposed to do so I can do it anyway," all done in the context of loving physical contact and laughing and tousling and great pleasure.

When we have enough of our sense of self, our survival system can integrate the differences that require us to respond to the outside as well as our inside world (our curious explorer system). We become members of our culture. The role-systems that develop are related to both the outside and the inside context and can continue to develop over time. Thus, in the process of being socialized (an ambivalent experience at best), there is a potentially reparative containment when we develop roles that work for us socially and that continue to develop as we develop. These inter-person roles respond to the goals of both our self and the context and contribute to both inner-person and system-as-a-whole as they develop.

Our compliant and defiant role-systems

Our stubborn role-system (see Figure 6.9) is a good example of a role-system container for the early conflicts we experienced between our child selves and those adults who had the job of socializing us. Originally, saying "no" both

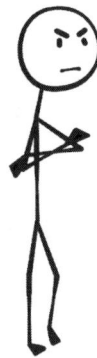

Figure 6.9

preserved our sense of self and signaled that we were not going to give up our integrity. In the best of worlds, during our terrible twos, saying "no" was both developmental and fun, similar to the five-year-old version described above. In contrast, in the worst of worlds it was experienced as a fight to the death. However, whereas in the past, stubbornness saved our life, in the present this same stubbornness prevents us from living it. As we say, there is no future in the past! When we are unaware of experiencing a threat in the present, we have no choice except to retreat into the survivor role-systems that we developed in the past. Past adaptive role-systems, like our stubborn compliant or defiant role-systems, were highly adaptive in containing threats when they were first developed but, unless they are updated, they are rarely useful in the present. Once again, threats in the real present need present solutions.

As we discussed in Chapter 5, we have a developing awareness of how we induce and are induced by role postures and how we unwittingly respond with role responses that were adaptive in the past but not useful in the present. Ducking our head in "obedient compliance" may have solved problems when we were three years old but will be costly to us when we are looking for a promotion at 33! Recognizing how our social role signals can induce old role responses from the past leaves us freer to respond with roles appropriate to the present.

When our social roles are driving forces

We negotiate our everyday lives using role-systems that develop from the inter-person system. Social roles are a compromise between the unconditional positive regard that nascent inner-person systems "know" intuitively is their birthright and the demands of the cooperation which is required to restore our birthright. When, as we described above with the small child, socializing role interactions also contain repairs (a restoration of attunement and resonance, communicated empathically), all is well and a developing context is restored. The advantage is that the system maintains a viable equilibrium and thus survives.

In addition to the influence of how social role-systems develop, it is important to recognize the context of the development of our social roles. For example, there is a story that Eskimo children are "shamed" by the village from the first time they move onto thin ice. In this case, the shame is life-saving. And the survivor goal is quite rightly given precedence over the developmental goal.

Summary

By observing the characteristics of our role-system behavior, we can surmise whether it will serve as a driving or a restraining force in relationship to its goals and to the goals of its larger context. Locating our role-system on the map will tell us where we are and "who" we are simply by observing the way we behave in our role! For example, if we are focusing on our self-development with curiosity, we are in a "developing" inner-person role that can lead to personal insight. If we have the same inner-person focus without curiosity, we are in our "closed" survivor role, safe from any personal insights! If we are in a "personalizing" role, are we trying to understand something about our own dynamics, or are we taking something "just personally" and feeling threatened or angry? The first would be an inner-person driving force towards self-development. The second would be a restraining force to self-development but a driving force in closing boundaries to threatening inputs that would otherwise destabilize our system.

Our next chapter describes other applications and innovations we have made in SCT as we have worked with our role-systems map and introduces our new phylogenetic role protocol.

Note

1 Neuroscience research is now starting to orient to the interpersonal space as an alternative to "individual-centric" approaches and instead towards seeing the brain in interaction rather than isolation, or as SCT says, seeing the inter-person system. Fortunately, the technology for inter-brain connectivity analysis is starting to emerge in functional neuroimaging. For example, Ray, Roy, Sindhu, Sharan, and Banerjee (2017) are working to effect a shift "from a focus on neural information contained *within* brain space to a multi-brain framework exploring degree of similarity/dissimilarity of neural signals *between* multiple interacting brains." This is exciting as it marks a potential shift to technology that can enable tracking more about the various system levels and particularly the similarity and differences in neural signals in functional subgrouping.

References

Badenoch, B. (2011). *The brain-savvy therapist's workbook*. New York, NY: Norton.

Badenoch, B. (2017). *The heart of trauma: Healing the embodied brain in the context of relationships (Norton series on interpersonal neurobiology)*. New York, NY: Norton.

Bowlby, J. (1969). Instinctive behavior: An alternative model. In *Attachment and loss: Vol. 1, attachment*. New York, NY: Basic Books.

Bowlby, J. (1979). *The making and breaking of affectional bonds*. London, UK: Tavistock.

Bowlby, J. (1982). *Attachment* (2nd ed.). New York, NY: Basic Books.

Bowlby, J. (1988). *A secure base: Clinical applications of attachment theory*. London, UK: Routledge.

Cozolino, L. (2010). *The neuroscience of psychotherapy: Healing the social brain* (2nd ed.). New York, NY: Norton.

Cozolino, L. (2012). *The neuroscience of psychotherapy: Building and rebuilding the human brain* (2nd ed.). New York, NY: Norton.

Cozolino, L. (2014). *The neuroscience of human relationships: Attachment and the developing social brain*. New York, NY: Norton.

Dikker, S., Wan, L., Davidesco, I., Kaggen, L., Oostrik, M., McClintock, J., . . . Poeppel, D. (2017). Brain-to-brain synchrony tracks real-world dynamic group interactions in the classroom. *Current Biology, 27*(9), 1375–1380. doi:10.1016/j.cub.2017.04.002

Gantt, S. P. (in press). Systems-centered theory (SCT) into group practice: Beyond surviving ruptures to repairing and thriving [special issue]. *International Journal of Group Psychotherapy*.

Gantt, S. P. (2018). Developing groups that change our minds and transform our brains: Systems-centered's functional subgrouping, its impact on our neurobiology, and its role in each phase of group development. *Psychoanalytic Inquiry: Today's Bridge between Psychoanalysis and the Group World [Special Issue], 38*(4), 270–284. doi:10.1080/07351690.2018.1444851

Gantt, S. P. (2019a). Implications of neuroscience for group psychotherapy. In F. J. Kaklauskas & L. R. Greene (Eds.), *Core principles of group psychotherapy: An integrated theory, research, and practice training manual* (pp. 156–170). New York, NY: Routledge.

Gantt, S. P. (2019b, February). *Seeing ourselves and our groups as living human systems: How systems-centered groups develop our minds and transform our brains*. Institute Opening Plenary presented at the American Group Psychotherapy Association Annual Meeting, Los Angeles, CA, US.

Gantt, S. P., & Agazarian, Y. M. (2010). Developing the group mind through functional subgrouping: Linking systems-centered training (SCT) and interpersonal neurobiology. *International Journal of Group Psychotherapy, 60*(4), 515–544. doi:10.1521/ijgp.2010.60.4.515

Gantt, S. P., & Agazarian, Y. M. (2011). The group mind, systems-centred functional subgrouping, and interpersonal neurobiology. In E. Hopper & H. Weinberg (Eds.), *The social unconscious in persons, groups, and societies: Volume 1: Mainly theory* (pp. 99–123). London, UK: Karnac Books.

Gantt, S. P., & Badenoch, B. (2020). Systems-centered group psychotherapy: Developing a group mind that supports right brain function and right-left-right hemispheric integration. In R. Tweedy (Ed.), *The divided therapist: Hemispheric difference and contemporary psychotherapy*. London, UK: Routledge.

Heard, D., & Lake, B. (1986). The attachment dynamics in adult life. *British Journal of Psychiatry, 149*, 430–439.

Heard, D., & Lake, B. (1997). *The challenge of attachment for caregiving*. London, UK: Routledge, Chapman & Hall.

Lewin, K. (1951). *Field theory in social science*. New York, NY: Harper & Row.

McCluskey, U. (2002). The dynamics of attachment and systems-centered group psychotherapy. *Group Dynamics: Theory, Research and Practice, 6*(2), 131–142. doi:10.1037/1089-2699.6.2.131

McCluskey, U. (2005). *To be met as a person: The dynamics of attachment in professional encounters*. London, UK: Karnac Books.

McGilchrist, I. (2009). *The master and his emissary: The divided brain and the making of the western world*. New Haven, CT and London, UK: Yale University Press.

Porges, S. W. (2007). The polyvagal perspective. *Biological Psychology*, 74(2), 116–143. doi:10.1016/j.biopsycho.2006.06.009

Porges, S. W. (2011). *The polyvagal theory: Neurophysiological foundations of emotions, attachment, communication, and self-regulation*. New York, NY: Norton.

Ray, D., Roy, D., Sindhu, B., Sharan, P., & Banerjee, A. (2017). Neural substrate of group mental health: Insights from multi-brain reference frame in functional neuroimaging. *Frontiers in Psychology*, 8, 1627. doi:10.3389/fpsyg.2017.01627

Schore, A. N. (2019a). *Right brain psychotherapy*. New York, NY: Norton.

Schore, A. N. (2019b). *The development of the unconscious mind*. New York, NY: Norton.

Chapter 7

Implications for practice from our role-systems map

Our role-systems map has proven very useful in helping us to identify criteria for assessing readiness to change. First, how we talk and how we behave locates us in our role-systems map, enabling us to connect the role output and goals to the source system's goals (as we discussed in Chapter 5). An important implication from this work is that by identifying the system, we have also identified parameters for assessing "readiness for change." For example, when we observe an inner-person closed "personal" role-system, we can assume that it is located in a closed survivor system and that readiness for change is low. Alternatively, if the personalizing system is also showing curiosity, we can locate our role-system in an open survivor system, indicating greater readiness for change. In addition, we can assess when the role-system being used is a driving or a restraining force to the goals of our context. In effect, our role-system signals the driving and restraining forces that let us know how ready we are for work in our context.

Using our role-systems map to assess readiness for change

Each of our three systems, inner-person, inter-person and system-as-a-whole, have specific criteria that identify those changes that can be integrated and those that cannot. Identifying the system that is active by its role-system output also allows us to identify what changes are within the systems' capacity. For example, if the role-system is identified as an inner-person survivor role-system, it is then important to assess whether it is a closed survivor system or an open survivor system. In the survivor roles of self-centered personalizing, the boundaries are closed to any input that is different from one's own. Until one can become curious (allow the life force to access the exploratory drive), it is impossible to change. Asking about curiosity tests the permeability of the role-system boundaries. A "curious" role behaves differently from a role that is not curious. The presence of curiosity signals an open survivor system, open to its curious explorer role. Curiosity indicates greater readiness for change. In contrast, readiness for change is low in the closed survivor system that is closed to its curiosity. The closed survivor system holds the goal of stability and resistance to change. Recognizing whether a person is curious will determine whether he or she is working within a closed or open system and, thus, his or her readiness for change.

These criteria link directly to our TLHS, which says that like any living human system, the survivor system survives and develops by integrating differences so that the system can develop from simpler to more complex and transform. In the process of developing and transforming, the survivor system boundaries open to the exploratory drive. This requires an explorer system with available curiosity as well as resonance to the closed survivor role. We know we are ready to change when our survival system has the energy of the exploratory drive to fuel it. In short, when we are curious, we can do the work to change. When we are curious, our boundaries are permeable, and we can move towards our developmental goals. When we are not curious, we remain behind closed boundaries. We survive but do not thrive.

Context, phase of development and readiness for change

For all three systems, readiness for change is also always determined by the phase of development of its context which, in turn, determines which restraining forces can be weakened without destabilizing the system. Being able to intuit the influence of the system-as-a-whole that elicits our role-system responses allows us to think about the influence of context. It is relatively easy to see what it is in the context of our experience that elicits our inner-person and inter-person role responses. Thus, by developing awareness of our own characteristic role locks in our responses, we can observe ourselves induced by or into the identified patient role in the context of the flight phase, to the scapegoat in the fight phase, sadistic or masochistic roles in the crisis of hatred, and merging or alienating roles in the intimacy phase. In SCT, it is important to see how our contexts are systems that generate and influence our role-systems and our readiness for change.

For example, when the context is the early flight phase, social roles in the inner-person system can be modified and anxiety-driving negative predictions can be undone. However, when in flight, the system is not ready to reduce outrage in the inner- or inter-person nor can inter-person anxiety yet be reduced. In fact, attempting to do so would be misattuned to the role-system context and, as with any misattunement, it would be likely to stimulate a more closed system.

Further, the example of a role of outrage is prototypical in the transition phase between flight and fight. An outrage role identifies either a closed inner-person survival system or a closed inter-person system role lock or both. The change map would take the route of crossing the boundary from survivor to curious explorer to curiosity about the inner-person context.

If this failed, the next step would be attuned subgrouping so that explorer energy is attuning to the survivor. If, on the other hand, the outrage was nested in an inter-personal subgroup, the route would be to arouse curiosity as to what in the context was being avoided by diversion from experiences of either rage or pain or grief.

An advantage of making this distinction is that it lets us know whether the role-system is or is not ready to change. When our role-systems are interactive, and we see, for example, attuned subgrouping, we can assume that these role-systems are outputs of the inter-person system, relating to inter-person goals. Recognizing the system-as-a-whole phase and its role-systems enables us to know what changes are possible, given the phase resources and its dynamics and what changes are not yet possible.

Survival system energy available for change

Another criterion for identifying when a role-system is ready for change requires recognizing when the person, subgroup or group is attuned to their survival system energies: their life force and their exploratory drive. Change requires both energies. In addition, the idea that change within a system can occur through changes within its role-systems introduces an even more challenging idea. As we noted in Chapter 6, this idea implies that role-systems as vectors can go both ways: they can serve as outputs from the system into the context and they can also serve as inputs to the role-system from the context.

When words don't cross the boundary

In our survivor roles of self-centered personalizing which contain resistance to change in the service of survival stability, our boundaries are closed to any input that is different from our own. Even attuned empathic words can fail to cross the boundary. Until we can become curious (allow the life force to access the exploratory drive), it is impossible to respond to someone except from our closed survivor role, much less change as the boundaries in closed past adaptive roles are impermeable to all differences. Understanding this is new to SCT practice and has some important implications. Curiosity fails when the survivor system is under threat. Thus, arousing curiosity when the survivor system is under threat fails more often than it succeeds! When words don't reach a patient, what will? SCT trusts that the averbal, limbic system–level human experience never closes. Thus, synchronized, resonant mirroring is a nonverbal communication at the autonomic nervous system level and is always a potential driving force at the wordless level in the *survival system*. SCT trains this level of reflection in its subgrouping process in the intimacy and work phases of development.

For example, in a conference large group that was working to recognize the whole group system voice in themselves, the group worked to explore dependency both in the authority phase and the intimacy phase:

> At one point, a member undid his judgments that had been blocking him from hearing the group voice in himself and discovered he was terrified at the edge of the unknown. The group initially found it hard to join this subgroup. One member joined with "scare" which was close enough to contain the member and the group. The next subgroup input had openness and freedom at the edge of the unknown. This was too different and the member holding the group's terror became more terrified. The leader and this member stayed in eye contact holding the terror together (an example of functional dependency), with the group silently supporting the work and many silently joining in holding the group's terror. Containing the annihilation anxiety at the edge of the unknown in nonverbal resonance was both moving and transformative for the member, the subgroup and the system–as–a–whole.
>
> (Gantt, 2016, p. 3)

This kind of resonant mirroring, of course, demands that therapists can access these steps in themselves. This is the rationale behind why developing access to the roles in the self is such a high priority in SCT training and also necessary if SCT practitioners are to internalize the values of humanizing, de-pathologizing, normalizing, legitimizing and universalizing.

Readiness in the context of the therapist/patient system

Lastly, a major goal in therapist–patient interactions in SCT is reinforcement of the open survivor self and arousal of curiosity in the inner-person system. Doing this depends on the context of the therapy system. Unless or until the patient, the therapist and the inter-personal system of therapist/patient are established, SCT assumes that no therapy can take place. This is the primary signal that the system contains readiness for change.

The additional step in SCT therapy is the establishment of working subgroups between the patient and therapist. One subgroup maintains the attachment behaviors communicated in resonance and attunement, and the other subgroup contains the inter-person empathic reality-testing role-systems in both patients and therapists and system-as-a-whole apprehensive intuitions. It is at the system-as-a-whole level that SCT assumes that the invisible systems of projective identification develop, intuitively sensed as a parallel process.

Projection is understood as the extrusion of a subsystem that serves as a containing role-system, the goal of which is to keep overwhelming differences contained within impermeable boundaries. In projective identification, a role-system develops in the system-as-a-whole between the sender and receiver.

As many of us know, the initial experience of a projective identification is almost intolerable to our inner-person system, but our inter-person system can develop tolerance for it. Thus, SCT views projective identification as a successful extrusion of an encapsulated subsystem from the patient into the containing system of the therapist. In the system-as-a-whole between the patient and therapist, it is the therapist who then does the work of integrating the difference, and when that has occurred, the system-as-a-whole changes and the patient is free to take a next step in their therapy. Thus, the therapist's readiness to integrate the difference is a signal for the readiness in the system-as-a-whole. This system dynamic applies both to the person system and to group systems. The dynamics of system encapsulation offer a system explanation for the preconscious and unconscious, as well as for the dynamics of repression and denial. In SCT, encapsulation is understood as a restraining role-system in relationship to system development goals, which becomes a driving force when the projective identification is integrated.

Training therapists

All of our new work started as we discovered our "mistake" in a training context. So it is fitting that we now come full circle to deepen our understanding of what is involved in training therapists (and likely attuned leaders and consultants). We have emphasized that the road to developing attunement begins at the edge of the unknown, where what we know is without words. In practice, from the early stages of systems-centered therapy, we have focused on undoing the anxiety that the unknown can generate. We have also conceptualized the unknown as the reservoir of all future knowledge which we apprehend without words before we can discover the words that help us to comprehend it. In our group and individual work, we encourage sitting with the chaos at the edge of the unknown, in spite of the fact that it can provoke not only anxiety, fear and/or dread but also annihilation anxiety. We also discovered that the more we are able to stay at the edge, the more likely we are to break through to a wordless understanding. Apprehension is different from comprehension. Exploring is not the same as explaining. Feeling is different from thinking.

Yet connecting attunement to empathy has some challenges. Some of these challenges are developmental and relate to modifying past role adaptations that blocked our development. Fundamental both in the training of SCT practitioners and also in the practice of SCT therapy is the ability to work towards establishing a climate of attunement and empathy. This requires training in theory but especially experiential training. SCT takes it for granted (as many therapies do) that nonverbal resonance is necessary (although not sufficient) if the goals of therapy are to be met. Developing the ability to be open to our own resonance and attunement is a challenge for all of us and beyond some of us. The question then arises as to how to train our SCT practitioners in this essential and transitional development.

Training for functional subgrouping

Not surprisingly, training for functional subgrouping is the major change process for both patients and practitioners in SCT and essential for practitioners in learning both resonant attunement and empathy. Reiterating the process of functional subgrouping:

> First, listen to what the other says. Then paraphrase both the other's words and the emotional music of the words that the other has said. This requires attunement and resonance with the other. Keep an eye on whether, as you are paraphrasing, the other shows non-verbally that they feel understood. If they keep a blank face, or look away, give the feedback that you have lost attunement with them. When the other says that they feel understood (and if you believe them through mutual resonance), prepare to separate. Note the transition from being joined in resonance and withdrawing your resonance and resonating with yourself. (At one point in time, you will discover frustration, grief and rage – before you accept the curiosity that goes with resonance with the self.) Once you have restored your resonance with yourself, open to whatever you discover you want to bring into the group and say "anyone else?" so that the other (or others) know that you have said enough of what you want to say and are ready to be paraphrased and reflected.

Functional subgrouping contains the potential for repairing our missed developmental steps and requires members to take their own time to integrate. For some it takes many years. For others, it is a good container for each appropriate developing step along the way. Functional subgrouping offers practice in separation and individuation in all the contexts where it has not yet happened and develops our capacity for regulating and co-regulating with others, which is our human preference (Porges, 1995, 2007, 2009, 2011) for managing the stress of the differences that are essential for human development.

Training for reality-testing

In training therapists, SCT also develops the necessary objective curiosity and reality-testing about whether the other is, in fact, in the same empathic resonance with you that you feel you are with them. Trainees learn how to check a mindread and observe nonverbal behavior to see whether it is congruent with one's impressions. Discovering the methods of curious objective observation can be as simple as requiring oneself to observe the behaviors that signal that the other is ready to hear you. (Observer training is built into learning to watch the faces in response to paraphrasing and reflecting in functional subgrouping; this develops the inter-person system.) A good way to develop this observational skill is to imagine that you are telling an actor how to copy the behaviors of a client who you feel is ready to hear you. This will require you to think and notice what "ready to hear you" behaviors look like, which may or may not be present when you feel that they are listening to you. For therapists familiar with the SAVI system for analyzing verbal interaction, the SAVI patterns of verbal behaviors can be used to identify and observe the role-system shifts and the different systems that are activating them.

The importance of training for reality-testing cannot be overemphasized. For example, when a leader diagnoses a group as "dead in the water," the diagnosis is often first made from the "feel" of the group energy and its impact on the energy of the therapist. Once the diagnosis is made, however, the questions in the therapist's mind have to do with checking whether or not their diagnosis is a projection or a perception. This takes reality-testing. Or is the group, in fact, integrating an experience after a fulcrum event and not "dead in the water" at all? If so, has the group just completed some inter-personal role-system work which will functionally result in group change? Or is the group angry with the therapist and members are in their inner-person role-systems, not knowing how to give voice to their experience (closed inner-person survivor role-system)? In this case, is the therapist able to scan for the data of how the role induction occurred? Was the therapist recently misattuned (a functional mistake), or has there been some earlier event that has not yet been surfaced and worked? Perhaps a structural event – like the therapist arriving at the group late!

Other trainees are not ready for this step, as they do not yet know the difference between what they feel and what they think. The first step then is to undo anxiety and the roles in which they are trapped in their inner-person system, as they try to do something they are not yet ready to do. With anxiety roles weakened and bypassed for the moment, the next step is to see whether, although blind to themselves, they can see the process in others. In other words, we try to mobilize the energy of their inter-personal system. If they can see the process happening outside themselves, they are much more likely to become curious and explore what it is inside themselves that enables them to see the difference. Recognizing this space inside themselves is a step towards affective attunement. As always, the first step in training is to become curious – does one know what attunement feels like? Can one notice when one is attuned and when one is not? This is a development within the inner-person system.

In training groups (and therapy groups), the method of functional subgrouping allows us to check out whether the other experiences us as attuned and empathic to them. It is in the intimacy phase of system development that explorations into one's own capacity for empathy is best explored because it is in this phase that the intensive work on separation and individuation is done. It does not matter whether one is experiencing the individual pleasure in merging, or the isolation of alienation, it is the shared attunement that allows one to shift from projection to perception. For example, a graphic experience of the difference between the realities of the inner-person survival system with its boundaries closed and the shared experience of resonance with others in a subgroup was voiced by one member in the alienated subgroup who burst out laughing, saying: "Here I am, cold and lost, floating in empty space, isolated, alone . . . in the middle of a whole subgroup of people who are sharing this same feeling of being alienated and alone!"

The experiential training our training groups provide is a key component in SCT training, as members learn to apply SCT first with themselves before using it with others. Exploring our new theory with our trainees has also been invaluable to us in developing SCT and most recently has led us to develop a new role protocol, our phylogenetic protocol.

A new protocol from role-system theory: phylogenetic protocol

Past role-systems developed as an adaptation to ruptures in our affiliation/attachment or in the conflict between our survival system dependence on affiliation/attachment and the demands that our significant others make when they socialize us (Twomey, Gantt, & Agazarian, 2006). Our basic role protocol is used in the authority phase of development where the work is to recognize one's closed role-systems. First, the person is asked to name the role and then explore and research how one thinks, feels, sees the world and relates to others from the role. Lastly, the work is to see how other's behaviors trigger our roles and our role-system behaviors trigger others.

Our "origin of role" protocol is not used until the intimacy or work phase where the tendency to blame the past has already been weakened by the work in the authority phase. In this role protocol, we have focused on the relationship between one's care-takers and oneself, using one's apprehensive memory of one's childhood experiences as the source of information. This leads to exploring one's "adapted" self in relationship to someone whose love was vital for one's feelings of well-being.

Our newest role protocol, which we are introducing here, recognizes not only that all past adaptations manage the conflicts between our affiliation/attachment dependence and socialization but that the adaptations happen in the context of historical influences in our family's past history that are implicit in our family's norms. This expands our orientation for framing the influence of the systems-as-a-whole that develop over time in the family's past history. By adding the dimensions of seeing the larger system context of the historical roots of our role-system development, we establish a system-centered perspective that frees us from taking our own role-systems just personally. SCT is reframing family norms in terms of the system-as-a-whole that develops not only in the family history but also in the past history of the family over generations.

SCT calls this new work our phylogenetic protocol. It has both some similarity, and some important differences, with the genogram used in some couples and family therapy. All families have a history; all families develop family norms influenced by past norms and imported into the present. Thus, the phylogenetic history of family norm formation is surfaced deliberately in SCT when there is readiness for change. The important SCT difference is that the SCT phylogeny protocol requires us to identify the influence of our early affiliation/attachment and social role-systems that we developed under the influence of the system-as-a-whole influences of our family norms. And in addition, this protocol provides a structure for looking at how these role-systems developed from the unique mix of our family's history of ethnicity, culture, religion, class, wealth, privilege, stereotypes, history and stories handed down through generations as each of these variables are established and/or modified. Reconceptualizing roles as systems in the context of their phylogeny is an important new method for resolving the pain, grief, rage and shame that are elicited when one fails to understand how old roles are adaptive, a failure that leads to taking our roles just personally. We recognized that some of the dimensions that influence the norms of all family systems are phylogenetic, developed over different generations and different cultures, unique to each family culture and general to all.

Working with our understanding of role-systems has enabled us to add this new role protocol, the phylogenetic protocol, to our existing role protocols. This new protocol has the goal of reorienting our relationship from only the personalized experiences of the dyadic role-systems of parent and child to our new understanding of roles as systems in the context of generations of family system norms. Thus, the phylogenetic protocol introduces the role-system-as-a-whole perspective to understanding the generational contextual influences on us of our family systems and is used in the work phase where the resources for seeing context are more developed.

The phylogenetic protocol orients us to how family norms-as-a-whole are handed down over generations, fluctuating in both traditional and/or non-traditional ways. Tracing the phylogeny puts the influences between parents and children along dimensions that are general to all family members (see Figure 7.1). For example, if a family has "come down in the world" this will have an impact on the goals that parents will have for the status of the marriage of their children. If the family has values around education, for a family member to decide whether or not to go to university will have an impact on the family norms with an impact that is more than just personal. It will also be both interpersonal and generational!

Becoming aware of the phylogenetic influences of family norms on the individual makes it difficult to take the influence of a single parent just personally as we view the perspective of the family system-as-a-whole over generations. Future work with the phylogenetic protocol will test out the impact of this new system's orientation on "not taking one's parents and their parenting just personally!"

Examples of some areas where family norms develop within the family system

Deviance: Differing from a norm or from the accepted standards of a society Families can be supportive of deviance, unsupportive of deviance, marginalize deviance, ostracize deviance, attack deviance. Family norms can be supportive of deviance like sexuality, ageism, cognitive deterioration, physical deterioration. Or family norms can institutionalize deviance like sexuality, ageism, cognitive deterioration, physical deterioration.

Ethnicity: Of or relating to large groups of people classed according to common racial, national, tribal, religious, linguistic or cultural origin of background. This includes ethnic minorities and ethnic enclaves [local, indigenous; old immigrant identity (European, Irish, Italian, Latino, Middle Eastern, Western Europe), recent immigrant, new immigrant].

Language Skills: No common language, poor language skills, medium language skills, fluent in new language.

Generation: All of the people born and living at about the same time, regarded collectively. This includes formal relatives: great grandparents or may also include those "married in," grandparents (potential 4 or more if including "married in"), parents (typically 2, yet often more with second or third or more marriages), or adopted relatives. Informal relatives: Unmarried "spouses," unrelated "in loco parentis," friends like family.

Gender: Patriarchy, bisexual, transgender, male-dominated, female-dominated. Gender refers to the socially constructed characteristics of women and men – such as norms, roles and relationships of and between groups of women and men. It varies from society to society and can be changed. While most people are born either male or female, they are taught appropriate norms and behaviors – including how they should interact with others of the same or opposite sex within households, communities and workplaces. When individuals or groups do not "fit" established gender norms they often face stigma, discriminatory practices or social exclusion – all of which adversely affect health. It is important to be sensitive to different identities that do not necessarily fit into binary male or female sex categories. Gender norms, roles and relations influence people's susceptibility to different health conditions and diseases and affect their enjoyment of good mental and physical health and wellbeing. They also have a bearing on people's access to and uptake of health services and on the health outcomes they experience throughout the life-course.

Profession/Work: Political (Democrat, Republican, other parties), professional or blue collar or entrepreneur (physician, lawyer, accountant, professor, educator, etc.), financers (bankers, brokers, big business), CEO, top manager, middle manager, and line manager.

Religion: Traditional, non-traditional, closed systems, open system religions. Old religions, traditional religions, religions organized around key religious leaders (Christianity, Buddhism, Muslim), non-traditional religions and cults.

Socio-economic Status: The rich, the poor, the mega-moneyed class, the professional class, the business class, the middle class, the working class, the lower class, the Romani, the homeless, itinerant workers, tramps, hobos.

Figure 7.1

This protocol is new for us, similar to earlier ones and different in important ways that are strengthening our capacity to see context. This takes us next to our first step in integrating our earlier work in SAVI with our role-system theory.

Back to our roots

Our role-system theory and its applications have led us full circle to where we started, that is, with the SAVI system for analyzing verbal interaction. Since SAVI enables mapping communication patterns as being entropic, neg-entropic or contingent, it can be used to diagnose the likelihood of a communication transferring information from one system to another (Simon & Agazarian, 1967, 2000). We discovered that visiting our role-system theory through the map of SAVI gives us another avenue for putting theory into practice.

Briefly, the SAVI Grid is a three-by-three Cartesian square. The first column relates to *person* or personal information. The second and third columns relate to *topic*. All communications can be coded as primarily topic-oriented (either factual or orienting) or person-oriented. The rows relate to the likelihood of the communication crossing the boundary and are labeled avoidance, contingent or approach. Avoidance outputs close boundaries in receiving systems and thus have a lower probability of crossing the boundary. Approach outputs have a better chance of crossing the boundary. Outputs in the contingent row are dependent on the larger communication context and can be used in the service of avoidance or approach.

As described in Chapter 5, we are now working with the idea of role-system output signaling both the origin of the role-system and the likelihood of the role-system output crossing the boundary into its target system. Linking to our newer theory, avoidance outputs in SAVI would also signal the origin of the role-system as a closed survivor role, while the approach outputs would signal an open boundaried role-system. This focus led us to realize that the SAVI Grid was a natural tool for expanding our way of thinking about recognizing role outputs not only by diagnosing them in terms of their originating system and goal but also in their potential for crossing the boundary. Serendipitously, this expands SAVI's application as a tool that can be used to identify role-system output from which one can then predict the originating system as well as the likelihood of information transfer.

We started first with our oldest SAVI illustrations and labeled this adaptation of the illustrated SAVI Grid as "Recognizing Roles" (see Figure 7.2). The illustrated coding categories seemed especially useful, as the illustrations seemed to capture some of the behavioral expression of the roles beyond the words even though SAVI actually codes verbal output.

Our second picture (see Figure 7.3) helped us go further in using the SAVI Grid to depict and potentially help us recognize our role-systems. This picture brings in more of the SAVI theory, and we found it even more useful. For example, in the avoidance row, the likelihood of information crossing the boundary is low as we typically fight over differences or use flight or competing roles to avoid differences. These three kinds of roles maintain the system in avoidance of information transfer and keep the

Recognizing Roles

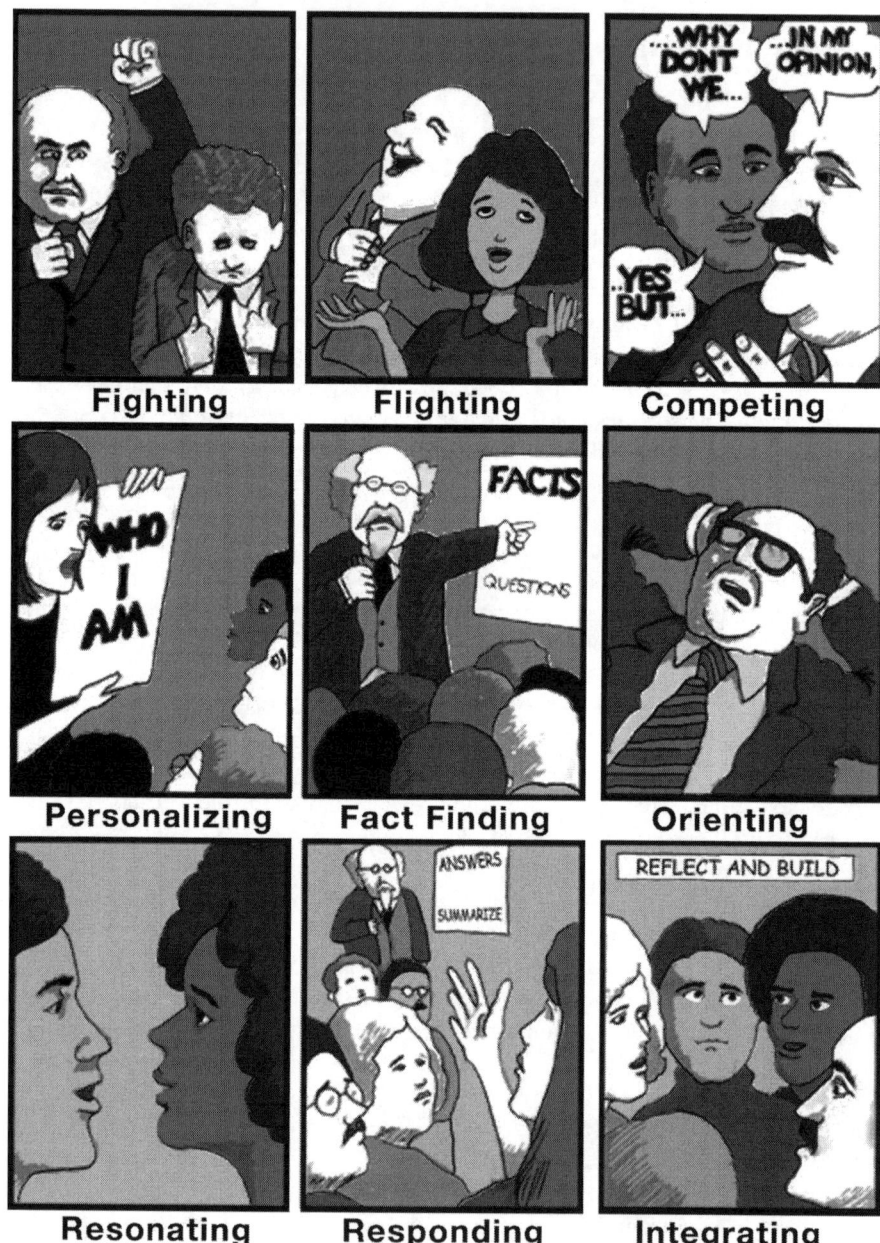

Figure 7.2

Recognizing Roles

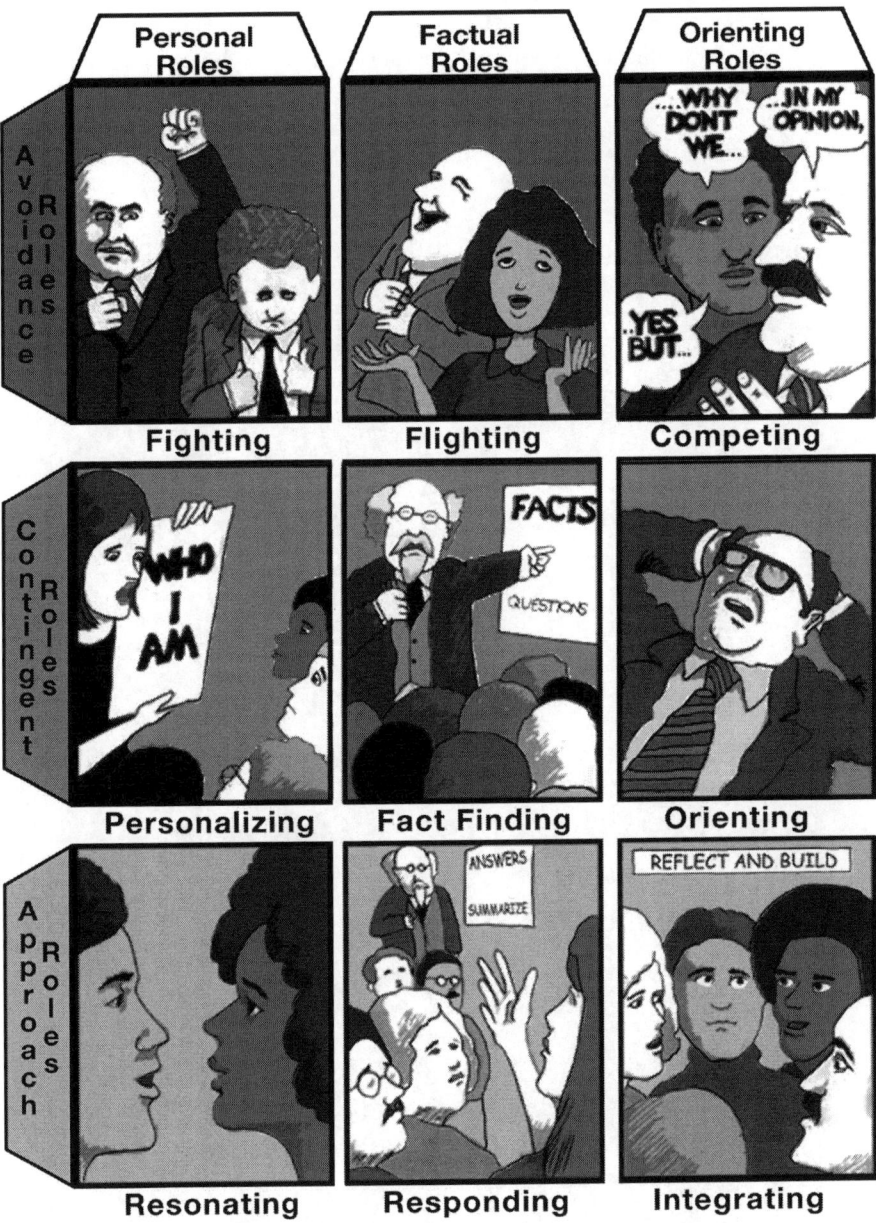

Figure 7.3

system in closed boundaries, staying safe. These roles that avoid communication or information transfer are closed survivor roles. In contrast, our approach roles have a much higher probability of information crossing the boundary, whether we are resonating or responding or integrating.

We can then start to look at SAVI patterns as a tool to diagnose an open or closed system in the inner-person or inter-person or the whole system (see Figure 7.4). This has been very exciting for us, and we are still exploring how we might use the SAVI patterns to identify and guide our work with role-systems. This is especially useful in our organizational work, as SAVI has easily crossed

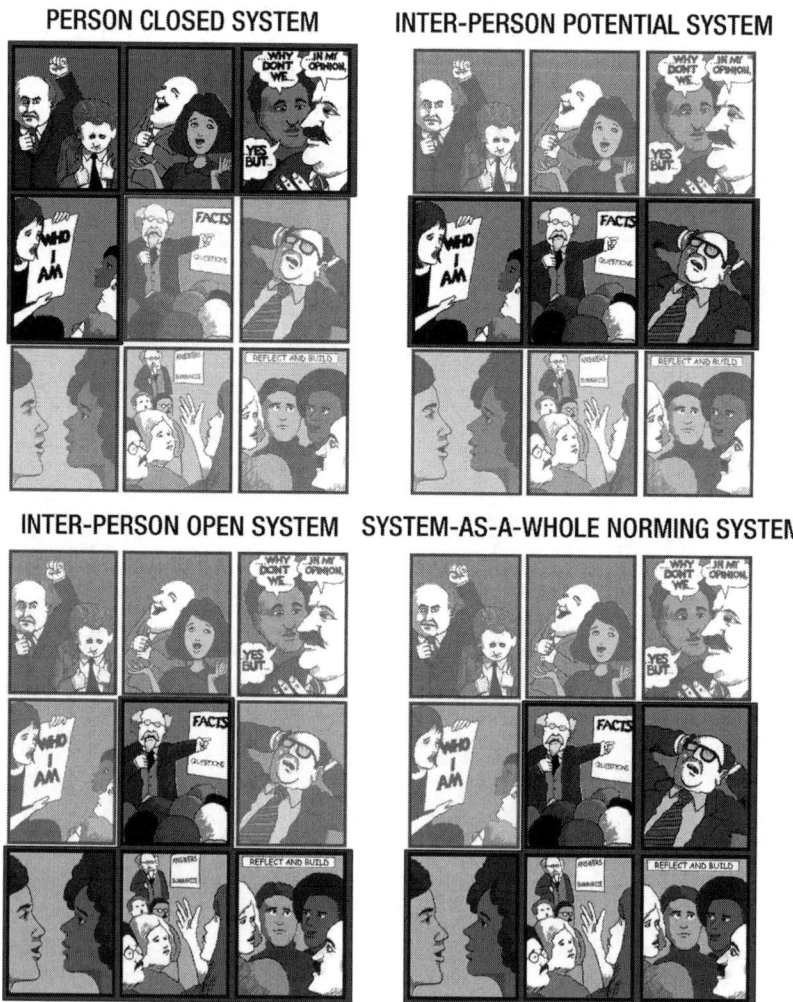

Figure 7.4

the boundary into organizations that want to improve communications. Linking SAVI patterns to role-systems may be a useful adjunct to working with teams in team development as the role-systems and their output identifiable in the SAVI Grid will also signal the phase of system development.

Summary

Integrating the role-system theory into our SCT practice has been exciting and is ongoing. This chapter has highlighted how our role-systems theory has deepened our capacity to assess readiness for change, essential for both clinical and organizational work. Our work with role-systems has also enabled a new role protocol (the phylogenetic protocol) that has proven useful to our clients in seeing themselves in context and lowering personalizing. Lastly, we presented how we are integrating our earlier work with SAVI with our role-systems map.

Our next chapter describes the important influences on SCT's model of phases of system development. Building on these, we then describe how we integrated these using SAVI and the force field to operationally identify and define each phase.

References

Gantt, S. P. (2016). A systems-centered perspective on two large groups. *Systems-Centered News, 24*(1), 2–3.

Porges, S. W. (1995). Orienting in a defensive world: Mammalian modifications of our evolutionary heritage: A polyvagal theory. *Psychophysiology, 32*(4), 301–318. doi:10.1111/j.1469-8986.1995.tb01213.x

Porges, S. W. (2007). The polyvagal perspective. *Biological Psychology, 74*(2), 116–143. doi:10.1016/j.biopsycho.2006.06.009

Porges, S. W. (2009). Stress and parasympathetic control. In L. R. Squire (Ed.), *Encyclopedia of neuroscience* (Vol. 9, pp. 463–469). Oxford, UK: Academic Press.

Porges, S. W. (2011). *The polyvagal theory: Neurophysiological foundations of emotions, attachment, communication, and self-regulation.* New York, NY: Norton.

Simon, A., & Agazarian, Y. M. (1967). *SAVI: Sequential analysis of verbal interaction.* Philadelphia, PA: Research for Better Schools.

Simon, A., & Agazarian, Y. M. (2000). SAVI: The system for analyzing verbal interaction. In A. Beck & C. Lewis (Eds.), *The process of group psychotherapy: Systems for analyzing change* (pp. 357–380). Washington, DC: American Psychological Association.

Twomey, H., Gantt, S. P., & Agazarian, Y. M. (2006). Roles. In S. P. Gantt & Y. M. Agazarian (Eds.), *Systems-centered therapy: In clinical practice with individuals, families and groups* (pp. 132–143). Livermore, CA: WingSpan Press. Reprint (2011). London, UK: Karnac Books.

Chapter 8

Theorizing about phases of system development

SCT identifies three overall phases of development: authority phase with its subphases of flight, fight, roles and role locks, and the crisis of hatred; intimacy phase; and work phase. In so many ways, Lewin's (1951) work has been the single most influential on SCT practice, and our work with phases is no exception. The influence of his force field model has enabled us to elucidate each of these phases (and subphases) of development as goal-directing systems that can be operationally defined as force fields of driving and restraining forces. The driving forces move the system in the direction of the developmental goal of the phase. The restraining forces orient to stability or survival.

This chapter describes the influences on our theorizing about phases and how we have used our systems theory and SAVI theory and grid in integrating these influences into our conceptualization of the phases of system development. We then elaborate our phase model and its applications in Chapter 9.

Other influences on SCT's theory and practice with phases

In addition to Lewin (1951), who has been the single most influential theorist for SCT, several theorists and practitioners have influenced us as we developed and applied systems theory to phases of development, most importantly the work of Bion (1961, 1963), Bennis and Shepard (1956) and Bridger (1987, 1990).

Bion

Bion (1961, 1963) worked in England with traumatized soldiers who had been sent home from the front to rehabilitate and return to fighting. Though the soldiers would proclaim wanting to improve to return to combat, their behavior suggested otherwise. Bion discriminated between implicit goals which can be inferred by behavior and explicit goals that are stated. From this recognition, Bion developed what he called the "basic assumptions" of group life that identify three implicit group goals: flight/fight, pairing and dependency.

He concluded that until these assumptions are worked through, the group or community will not be able to meet its explicit goals.

Influenced by Bion, SCT has adopted this discrimination between explicit and implicit goals. Both groups and members have goals that are explicit goals that can be stated. Groups and members, however, often behave quite differently from the goals that are stated. In understanding this, we have found it useful to intuit the implicit goals: the goals that are implied by what groups are doing rather than what they are saying they are doing.

Our pathway from Bion to applying systems theory to phases of development

What is easily compatible between Bion (1961, 1963) and systems thinking is that he arrived at his assumptions by observing the group-as-a-whole. In other words, in systems language, he observed the system and contrasted the relationship between the different member systems and the groups' systems. Thus, Bion's work was the forerunner of what systems-centered theory now takes for granted: that the implicit goals of members' role-system behaviors (like flight or fight role-systems) will be the major determinant of how members behave in a group, not their explicit or conscious goals (see Figure 8.1).

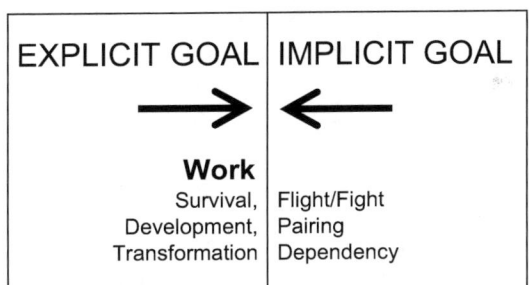

Figure 8.1

These role-systems are elicited by the group system. Thus, the implicit role inductions of the group system goals are the major determinate of group role behavior and not the personal goals of the members! Implicit group goals generate members' apparently "out of context" behavior at the cost of the explicit goals. This is where understanding isomorphy has been so useful for us.

For psychodynamic groups, the implicit can be framed as whatever the member's individual preconscious or unconscious goal might be. One can surmise in Bion's groups that the implicit goal was to *avoid* going back to the front lines. This contrasts with the soldiers stating that they wanted to return predominantly because of the explicit norms of the culture at that time in history or because of personal or family norms which meant they thought they *ought* to return to the fighting.

Integrating Lewin's (1951) observations of system output as signaling the groups' goals with Bion's (1961, 1963) work on implicit goals was very useful to us. SCT could then apply the Lewinian force field to determine how much energy is available for work by identifying the balance of driving and restraining forces in relationship to the group goals (see Figure 8.1). When the implicit and explicit goals are compatible, it is probable that both goals will be met. When, however, the implicit and explicit goals vector in different directions, it is likely there will be insufficient energy available for work towards its explicit goals. This simple formulation accounts for much of the frustration experienced in groups when the group "wants" to work but cannot. In SCT groups, subgrouping around the conflict between the driving and restraining forces has led the group to significant insight into the power of the implicit goals in the unconscious and preconscious. It has also been very useful in SCT groups to infer the implicit goal from the restraining forces of the group's force field. Surfacing implicit goals has enabled our groups to explore them and to weaken the relevant restraining forces.

Translating Bion's (1961, 1963) basic assumptions into systems language, it can be said that the implicit goals of flight/fight, pairing and dependency are restraining forces to the explicit goals of work. Work is defined by SCT as both the primary developmental goals of survival, development and transformation and also the secondary work goals that the group explicitly states (see Figure 8.1). The work in therapy groups, for example, is to understand and resolve conflicts, come to terms with reality, and transform human euphoria and anguish into normal human experience. The work in teams is to work together to use the resources of the team members to meet the goals of the team.

Bennis and Shepard

Another major influence on SCT's work with phases of system development are Bennis and Shepard (1956), who pioneered research and theory about group phases. Bennis and Shepard collected their data over a five-year period of observations of group development courses with graduate students in their university meeting as a group to "improve the internal communication system of the group" (Bennis & Shepard, 1956, p. 415). While observing their groups, they used Bion's (1961, 1963) theory to track the developmental process, leading to their identifying a predictable sequence in which the basic assumptions emerge. This major contribution introduced group phases into the group literature as they identified a predictable sequence in which Bion's basic assumptions emerged.

Bridger

Yvonne's work with Harold Bridger's workshops in the 1990s reinforced her orientation to group-as-a-whole goals and specifically phase of development goals. Bridger (1987, 1990), in what he called the double task of a group, emphasized the importance of having clear explicit goals for a group, without which, he claimed, the process tasks made it impossible for groups to direct their energy towards explicit goals. He also emphasized the importance of working with the underlying process in organizations as essential work so that the organization could meet its primary task. Thus, an important question from an SCT therapist when a group is in a muddle is to ask: "what is the group's goal right now?"

Other influences on SCT's understandings of phases

As we worked to formulate and implement our theory of phases, there were other significant influences on Yvonne and many of us working with her. Some of these as described here are quoted or drawn from both published and unpublished work from Yvonne's earlier writings about these influences, allowing us to include her voice in this chapter even though she died before it was written.

Tavistock

In the 1990s, it was Tavistock that gave me (Yvonne) invaluable training in group dynamics. In these trainings, I experienced firsthand how chaotic and disorganized the groups often became with members who were frequently overwhelmed by their emotional responses, some to the point of psychotic episodes in the workshops (Agazarian & Gantt, 2000). These experiences influenced us in SCT as we came to the conclusion that the chaos in these groups, from a group development frame, was the result of the groups being precipitated into their authority issue without the necessary preparation for containing and learning from human happiness and unhappiness.

Pat de Maré

For Yvonne, an important theoretical companion and influence was Pat de Maré. As Yvonne wrote in her foreword to *Small, Large and Median Groups* (Lenn & Stefano, 2012), "Pat . . . transformed the understanding of hatred in groups from a destructive affect into a natural, inevitable response to frustration, an energy that carries high potential for both destructive and constructive transformation." Continuing, Yvonne wrote:

> Much of our attitude towards human aggression is generated by our disapproval of it, and our disapproval is directly related to our superego fear of our unconscious potential. There is no question that we owe a great debt to Freud for his gift to us of the unconscious. But his gift came at

a price. Superego pathology has long been connected to a nightmare of demonic ideas, colluding with the profound fear of the unconscious that is inevitable if the unconscious is to contain Thanatos as well as Eros. What is more, the common psychodynamic understanding of hatred is closely linked to the destructive superego and superego guilt. Freud claimed that the energy of the superego is derived from the id. It is at this theoretical point that Pat introduced a seminal difference. Pat's argument (that might well turn the world of psychology upside down) is that the energy of the superego is not derived from the id, nor is it biological, nor is hatred and superego guilt a necessary corollary. Whilst love *is* linked to Eros, hate *is not* linked to Thanatos. "Hate is not the adversary of Eros but the inevitable irreversible outcome of the frustration of Eros: if there is any adversary to Eros, it is . . . ananke . . . external necessity."

Thus, Pat transforms Freudian pessimism into optimism by reversing Freud's thesis that civilisation is built upon the passive renunciation of instinctual gratification. On the contrary, says Pat, "it is the active frustration of hate to which the evolution of culture owes it origins . . .". Whereas, for Freud, the solution is passive, for Pat it is active. "It has become . . . clear to us that hate, arising out of the frustrating situation of the larger group . . . provides the incentive for dialogue and becomes transformed, through dialogue, into the impersonal fellowship of Koinonia . . ."

In the meantime, however, we in the field of psychotherapy are living under the tyranny of the superego. Perhaps the most destructive misunderstanding is to fail to see the difference between superego pathology and normal human aggression. Human aggression is the potential energy fundamental to fueling the flow of energy and information between all levels of human exchange. It is also the potential energy necessary to manage the inevitable frustrations that occur in everyday life. It is only when normal human aggression is viewed through the lens of the punitive superego that it becomes pathological.

All in all, the contribution of Pat's that has the most impact on me and, indeed, perhaps on the conductors and leaders of groups in the future, is his reinterpretation of superego hatred into the raw material for creative energy. Many groups live with the terrible consequences of misunderstanding hatred as if it is linked to human aggression, and linking the two give both a bad name. Framing as pathological what could be otherwise interpreted as normal human conflict has important clinical consequences. For example: the exogenous depression that comes from people turning the other cheek and turning their aggression back in on themselves; the superego criticism of sadism and masochism that prevents the conflicts that they contain to be explored without judgment; the "anger management techniques" that teach people to act nicely instead of acting out, without understanding that it is not just their angry hatred that is being modified but also their living energy. Perhaps most serious of all is the acquired fear of aggression. Fear of aggression goes hand in hand with fear of feeling, and fear of feeling is too often resolved by rationalisation. It might be common knowledge, but perhaps not common understanding, that feelings feel the same whether they are generated by thoughts or whether generated by our basic sensory experience of the world. From this confusion, communication norms develop that are manifested in anxiety-laden explanations of the past or present, repetitive stories about childhood, and a basic split between good and evil. When perception is based on projection, people become enmeshed in the anguish of personalising.

In summary, Pat's work [has been] ground-breaking and mind-blowing, [and for us] has had enormous implications for [our] management of hatred in groups . . . Pat's single, significant reframing of the understanding of the dynamics of aggression and hatred . . . might permanently change the practice of group.

(Agazarian, 2012, pp. xxi–xxiii)

Yvonne goes on in a footnote to write:

Pat is not alone in understanding that metabolizing hatred into fellowship results in a different potential for communication. Bennis and Shepard (1956) translated Bion's basic assumptions into a group development model that is not included in the Foulksian tradition. They then defined the common group eruptions of hatred towards the leader as a barometric event that generated the transition from preoccupations with authority into the phase of intimacy. In my turn, I then translated their developmental model into a systems approach, calling their fulcrum event "the crisis of hatred," common to the development of all isomorphic systems, whether the system be the person, member, sub-group, or the group-as-a-whole.

(Agazarian, 2012, p. xxiii)

Earl Hopper

Earl has been another important friend and theoretician interested in systems and a "comrade" who supported and influenced SCT and Yvonne and Susan's work. His theoretical conversations with Yvonne were important in our theorizing. We quote here the links that Yvonne made between SCT's phases and Earl's work written on the occasion of Earl's book *Traumatic Experiences in the Unconscious Life of Groups* (Hopper, 2003):

Earl Hopper, in his important, profound and well reasoned book, introduces a fourth basic assumption (incohesion) to the three basic assumptions (flight/fight, pairing and dependency) introduced by Bion. Hopper's theory of incohesion provides us with a new way of thinking about annihilation anxiety, which he discusses in terms of the unconscious fears of annihilation connected to the fears of separation.

In his theory of incohesion: aggregation/massification, Hopper identifies encapsulation as a major defense against annihilation (related to
traumatic experiences around separation). What is encapsulated is the
unconscious fear of annihilation and the oscillation between the fission and
fragmentation associated with contact-shunning, and the fusion and confusion associated with merger-hunger. Encapsulation dynamics contribute
to the formation of the personal roles of crustacean and amoeboid, and the
social dynamics of aggregation and massification . . .

Earl Hopper defines incohesion as an interaction of inter- and intra-
personal processes within a wider trans-generational social context. (A
cousin, perhaps, to SCT's construct of the pervasive transference.) He
summarizes his theory of incohesion as a universal sequence beginning
with traumatic events (involving loss, abandonment and damage) followed
by fears of annihilation and separation which give rise to intra-psychic
oscillations. These oscillations occur between processes that he calls fission and fragmentation on the one hand, and fusion and confusion on the
other, related to the lost or damaging object.

Fission and fragmentation are manifested in what he calls aggregation
in persons and society which are neither interdependent, nor in sympathy
with one another (a group of the alienated?). Fusion and confusion are
manifested in what he calls massification where there is a maximal degree
of mutual attraction based on illusion and without interdependence or
sympathy with one another (a group that is enchanted and merged?). We
in SCT would ask whether the common factor is the absence of attunement, empathy and resonance within, between and among people in
both subgroups.

Hopper states that the intra-psychic oscillation between these two
states is defended against by encapsulation, a process that attempts to survive the introjected object which is experienced as a foreign body in the
psyche. Disassociations from the encapsulation become contained in character formations (SCT would probably identify them as roles) which he
calls crustacean and amoeboid. The crustacean is contact-shunning and is
characterized by the fission and fragmentation of aggregation. The amoeboid is merger-hungry and is characterized by the fusion and confusion of
massification.

What we may learn most from reading Hopper's profound thinking presented in this surprisingly readable book is how he makes the bridge from
his theory to the treatment of difficult patients. He identifies aggregation
and massification as a characteristic of regressed groups. In groups of the
traumatized, however, where survivor guilt, and perhaps more important,
survivor shame underlies the suffering, aggregation and massification are
likely to be chronic.

Hopper discusses three of his groups, which communicate the dedication he has to his theory and the attunement he has with the unconscious

that his theory reveals. In the first two groups, he explores the two different characterizations or crustacean and amoeboid characteristics (two different members who typify the roles) within the context of a group-analytic group in which he frames his associative interpretations to the group process to the deep primal responses to separation and trauma. His examples are particularly illustrative by his focus on the group's reactions to separation as they prepare for his absences.

In his discussion of the third group he makes a cogent and moving argument for applying the principles of his basic assumption about incohesion to survivors of trauma, enabling them to survive anew the pain of annihilation anxiety, survival guilt, and, as he says, most importantly, survivor shame. Most moving, is his understanding that because of the shame of being abused, it is important to work the traumas in homogenous groups.

Where Hopper's theory of incohesion complements our thinking is in a deeper understanding of the dynamics of the phase of intimacy. We explain the splitting that occurs in the intimacy phase in terms of the vicissitudes of discrimination and integration in the process of separation and individuation: attributing separation to discriminating differences in the apparently similar and individuation to discriminating similarities in the apparently different. The deeper, psychodynamic experiences of alienation we explain in terms of a barrier experience in which there is a primary split between good and bad which makes it impossible to discriminate the good in the bad or the bad in the good. Thus the emergence of the roles characterized either by alienation and blind despair or by merging and blind hope.

Where Hopper is importantly different in his approach is that both his thinking and his interpretation to group and individual dynamics is deeply related to the personal and social unconscious, whereas ours are related to the development of apprehensive containment that enables the individual and the group to discover titrated layers of unconscious material. Hopper's work is particularly important for us in SCT as it is an extraordinarily readable representation of how one thinks, and how one interprets group and individual dynamics that exist at a deeper level of unconsciousness than those addressed by either Freud or Klein.

Hopper's incohesion dynamics are pre-splitting and related to universal human principles of annihilation anxiety, which he discusses in terms of the deeply unconscious fears of annihilation connected to the fears of separation. For our SCT group members it will be interesting to explore the similarities and the differences between Hopper's understanding of the fears of annihilation around separation with the experiences that occur for us as we continue to surface deeper and deeper levels of the unknown in the process of transformations.

(Agazarian, 2003, pp. 3–4)

All of these influences have been quite important either in developing our SCT phase model or in deepening our understanding of phase dynamics. Their impact helped lay the foundation for our own work of applying our TLHS to phases of system development and our deepening understanding of the phase dynamics for all living human systems.

Formulating the phases of system development

In spite of the enormous impact these theorists, practitioners, friends and colleagues had on our work with phases of development, it was in applying our systems theory that our systems phase model fully came to life. Turning to our own systems theory and methods enabled us to deepen our understanding of phases of system development as we developed operational definitions of the phases and how to influence phase dynamics towards development by introducing a systems way of working with group phases.

Using SAVI to recognize individual and group communications

Our early work with the SAVI system for analyzing verbal interaction had enabled us to code communication patterns in a person or in a larger system. This was very helpful, as it enabled us to see communication patterns at different system levels (see Chapters 4 and 7). To recap, SAVI (Agazarian, 1968; Simon & Agazarian, 1967, 2000) was developed as an operational definition of Shannon and Weaver's (1964) mathematical theory of communication: they identified an inverse relationship between entropic noise in the communication channel and the probability that the information in the communication will be transferred. The SAVI Grid enabled coding communication behaviors that are likely to transfer information (neg-entropic) as well as identifying those that are unlikely to transfer information (entropic). This coding system can be used to code communication patterns in a person or that of a larger system.

Using SAVI enabled us to "hear" the group-as-a-whole communication output, as well as discern the outputs for the individual members and the group's subgroups and to assess the probability that the communications are in the direction of the therapeutic or developmental goals or are entropic and more oriented to survival goals. SAVI can also be used in diagnosing the relationship between the driving and restraining forces to communication: communications that demonstrate the likelihood of transfer of information qualify as approach behaviors that move the system towards the goal, and those that interfere with the transfer of information qualify as avoidance and move the system towards the implicit goals of flight, fight or freeze.

The SAVI system for analyzing verbal interaction (Simon & Agazarian, 1967) uses trained coders to categorize the verbal behaviors (every three seconds), for example, self-criticism, thinking out loud or intellectualization. We could then identify communication patterns that showed differential frequencies of approach or avoidance behaviors for different phases of development and recognize distinctive communication patterns in each phase of development. For example, in the grid that we linked to the flight phase (see first picture in Figure 8.2), the SAVI coded behaviors that occurred in each square of the SAVI grid are identified by a box drawn around the behavior. Also in Figure 8.2, the second flight SAVI grid elaborates and shows the frequency in which these behaviors occur. In the avoidance row, flight is characterized by higher frequencies in "factual avoidance" (flight) and "orienting avoidance" (obscurity). Tallying the number of coded behaviors in the different classes yielded visual patterns of the relative use of driving or restraining communications; for example, personal message/avoidance does occur in square one, yet as it shows in the second picture in Figure 8.2, these are lower-frequency behaviors. These SAVI grids of the phases were identified by matching the SAVI patterns to the predictable communications in the different phases. These three figures show the patterns in flight (Figure 8.2), fight (Figure 8.3) and the barometric event or crisis of hatred (Figure 8.4). (Note: the contingent classes are reserved for those codes which can be driving or restraining dependent upon whether they are followed by a driving or a restraining force.) Thus, by analyzing the communication patterns in the group it became possible to diagnose the phase in which the group was working and to operationally define each phase by its communication patterns.

SAVI was also useful for comparing the group-as-a-whole pattern of communication with the patterns of the individual members. In one study, Yvonne

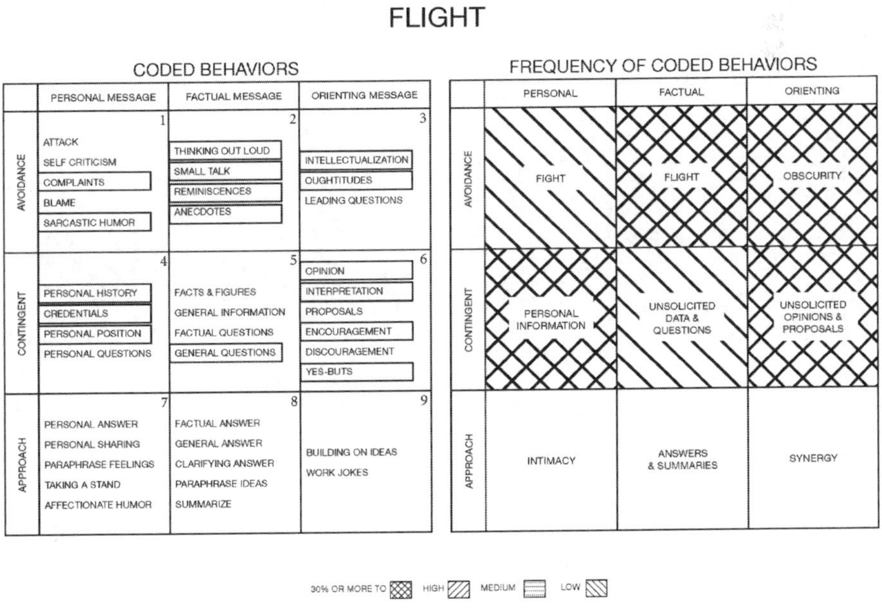

Figure 8.2

FIGHT

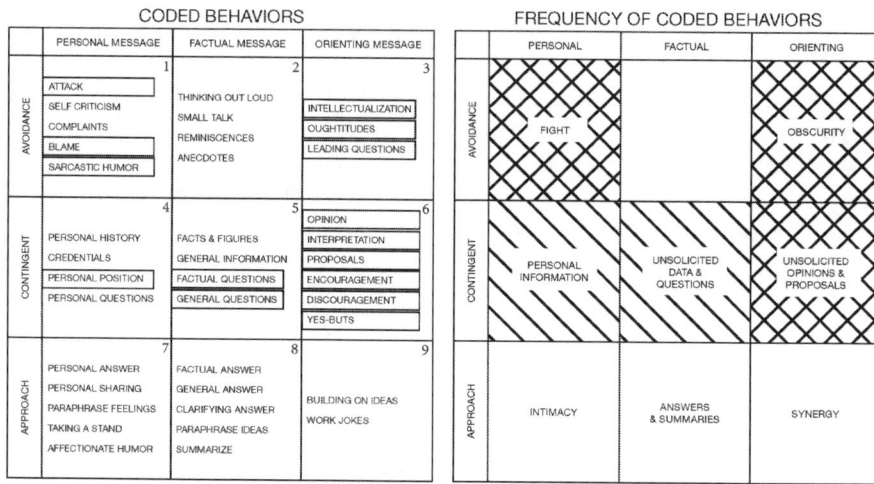

Figure 8.3

BAROMETRIC EVENT

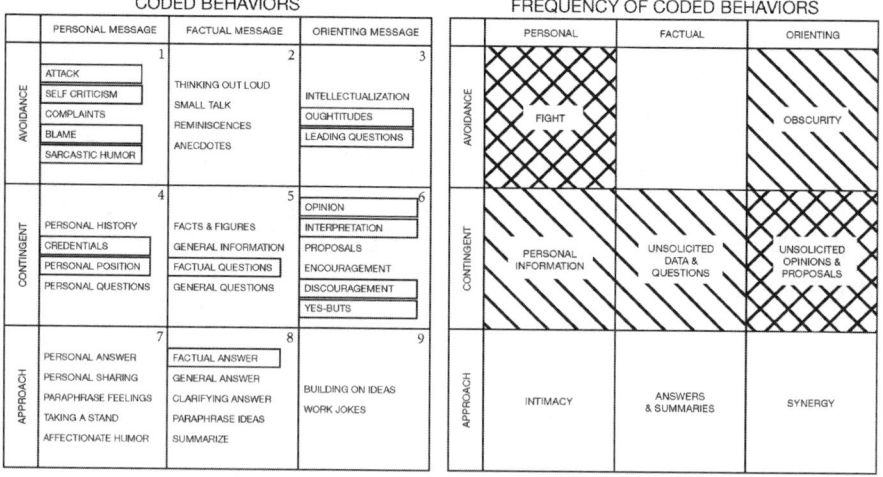

Figure 8.4

and Anita Simon first coded the whole group session in SAVI, then divided it into quartiles and coded the central ten minutes of each quartile. This made it possible to compare the quartile patterns with the pattern of the group-as-a-whole. There was negligible variance between the quartile patterns and negligible variance between the quartile patterns and the pattern of the group-as-a-whole. However, when the patterns of the individual members in each quartile were coded, there was considerable variance. Something was maintaining the group flight communication pattern in spite of the fluctuating patterns of the individual members (Agazarian & Gantt, 2000).

This raised an important question. If the group patterns were the same and the individual patterns were different, how did the group system pattern remain the same? What happened to wash out the variability? On closer inspection, it became clear what was happening: the group pattern was maintained in that whenever one individual would introduce driving forces, another would introduce restraining forces. Thus, in each segment, the system was stabilized in flight. What is more, it was not possible to predict which particular member would introduce restraining forces. In one surprising section, members contributed to a driving pattern, and it was the group therapist who introduced a restraining force which reinstated the flight! This informal research strongly supported the SCT idea that it is the system that has a greater influence on communication than the subsystems of its members.

These findings could not be attributed simply to group norms. If it was a matter of group norms, individuals would be specifically influenced towards predictable communication patterns throughout the development of the group. Instead, what actually happened was that different individuals made the inputs that maintained the pattern. These findings supported our hypothesis that the communication norms change as the phases of development change. Thus, even the work pattern of a "working" group will almost certainly be redirected into flight when, for example, at the threshold of new work, the group is at the edge of the unknown and becomes anxious.

Integrating the force field with our SAVI map

Returning to the force field to map the conflict between the forces that drive towards the goal and those that restrain the drive, we reframed the approach and avoidance categories in the SAVI map as a force field (just as we did with noise and clear communication in Chapter 2). Observing the SAVI force field for each phase of development made it possible to use SCT to identify which particular restraining forces to weaken within each phase in order to release the developmental drive. This leads us to our next step, identifying the restraining forces specific to each phase of development and how to weaken them to release the driving forces towards work.

For example, in the flight phase (see Figure 8.5), avoidant restraining forces are predominantly ambiguity or redundancy, whereas approach driving forces give evidence that communication has crossed the boundaries (for example, building on another's idea with specificity or getting to the bottom line).

FLIGHT

Driving →	← Restraining
Building with specificity → on another's idea	← Ambiguity
Getting to the bottom → line	← Redundancy

Figure 8.5

On the other hand, depressive restraining forces (turning retaliatory impulses back on the self) characterized the transition between the flight and fight subphase (see Figure 8.6), and despair (denial of hope for change) characterized the alienation subphase in intimacy.

TRANSITION TO FIGHT

Driving →	← Restraining
Undoing boomerang & → exploring retaliatory impulse	← Turning retaliatory impulse back on the self in boomerang

Figure 8.6

As all groups are capable of "hopping" from one phase to another as different subgroups surface, SCT diagnoses the overall phase of the group by observing the communication pattern that is emerging from the whole group system. This is similar to how SCT diagnoses role-systems from the communications and behaviors that emerge from the members, as we discussed in Chapter 7. From a systems perspective, the output of the group system is a useful indicator of the way information is organized within the whole system and at each system level. These identifiable patterns of organization reflect the group phase. Thus, the communication pattern is a more reliable indicator of "what" the group is doing than what the group "says" it is doing, similar to Bion's (1961, 1963) implicit and explicit goals. Also, drawing from Festinger (1953), how a group functions is a consequence of its process of communication (Gantt & Agazarian, 2007, p. 257). SCT now applies this to looking at the phase-specific pattern of communication of each system in the hierarchy of role-systems, each of which can be defined as a force field of driving and restraining forces that approach or avoid the developmental goal of the phase. Most SCT practitioners use a working knowledge of SAVI to guide their recognition of the system's phase of development as phase recognition is essential for SCT leaders.

We have included a section from our original phase chart that shows the subphases in the authority phase (see Figure 8.7) and the restraining forces for

SCT® MODIFICATIONS OF RESTRAINING FORCES TO GROUP DEVELOPMENT

The chart below displays the forces that restrain the spontaneous drive towards system development. Column one displays the core conflict in each phase of system development. Column two displays the specific restraining forces that impede development of the individual system. Column three displays the symptoms generated by the conflicts that are modified when the restraining forces are reduced.

PHASE ONE OF GROUP DEVELOPMENT: AUTHORITY		
FLIGHT SUBPHASE Impulse to contain dependency in the identified patient.	**SOCIAL DEFENSES** Stereotypic social communication.	Inauthenticity.
	THE TRIAD OF SYMPTOMATIC DEFENSES 1. Anxiety-provoking thoughts, ruminations and worrying that divert attention from reality-testing.	Anxiety.
	2. Tension-generating stress-related psychosomatic defenses which avoid the experience of emotion.	
TRANSITIONAL SUBPHASE BETWEEN FLIGHT AND FIGHT Impulse to target differences.	3. Defending against the retaliatory impulse by constricting it in depression or discharging it in hostile acting out.	Masochistic depression. Sadistic & hostile acting out.
FIGHT SUBPHASE Impulse to discharge hostility through scapegoating.	**ROLE LOCK DEFENSES** (interdependence of roles) Creating one-up/one-down role relationships like identified patient & helper; scapegoat & scapegoater; defiant & compliant.	Reciprocal maladaptive role pairing & role induction.
TRANSITIONAL SUBPHASE BETWEEN AUTHORITY AND INTIMACY Crisis of hatred, impulse to target authority.	**RESISTANCE TO CHANGE DEFENSES** 1. Externalizing conflicts onto those in authority: defensive stubbornness & suspicion from the righteous & complaining position.	Blaming authority for all problems.
	2. Disowning authority: defensive stubbornness & suspicion of self that blames personal incompetence.	Blaming self for all problems.
PHASE TWO OF GROUP DEVELOPMENT: INTIMACY (creating interdependence in relationships)		
ENCHANTMENT AND HOPE SUBPHASE Impulses to idealize the group and create a cult.	**DEFENSES AGAINST SEPARATION** Enchantment, idealization, blind trust of others, merging & love addiction as defenses against differences.	Dependency at the expense of interdependence & exploitability.
DISENCHANTMENT AND DESPAIR SUBPHASE Impulses to alienate self in existential despair.	**DEFENSES AGAINST INDIVIDUATION** Disenchantment & blind mistrust of self, others & groups. Alienation, contempt & despair as a defense against similarities.	Independence at the expense of functional dependency & interdependence.
PHASE THREE OF GROUP DEVELOPMENT: INTERDEPENDENT (see here) LOVE, WORK & PLAY		
ONGOING PHASES OF WORK IN THE EXPERIENCED GROUP Failures in response to the role, goal and context.	**DEFENSES AGAINST KNOWLEDGE** Defenses against inner reality & comprehensive & apprehensive knowledge.	Impairment of decision making & implementation abilities. Loss of common sense & humor.
	DEFENSES AGAINST COMMON SENSE Defenses against outer reality & reality-testing.	Self-centeredness at the expense of both self & the environment.

Developed by Yvonne M. Agazarian (2008).

© 2020 Systems-Centered Training & Research Institute, Inc.

SCT® and Systems-Centered® are registered trademarks of the Systems-Centered Training and Research Institute, Inc., a non-profit organization.

Figure 8.7

group development that manifest as defenses at the individual level and show as symptoms or system output. This was our first force field on phases, though it did not yet include the driving forces, nor did we fully frame it in systems language. Rather, this first chart built a bridge for us between the psychodynamic language of symptoms and the systems language of restraining forces. And it importantly contained the idea that modifying restraining forces also altered the symptom output and led to group development.

Our later drawings made the force field (see Figure 8.8) even more explicit, as we returned to our circle or Lewinian "egg" to represent the system phase. Operationally defining each phase of system development as a force field then provides a map for therapists and leaders to guide their interventions towards weakening the phase–relevant restraining forces. This makes it less likely that leaders will push the group to do work it does not yet have the resources to do.

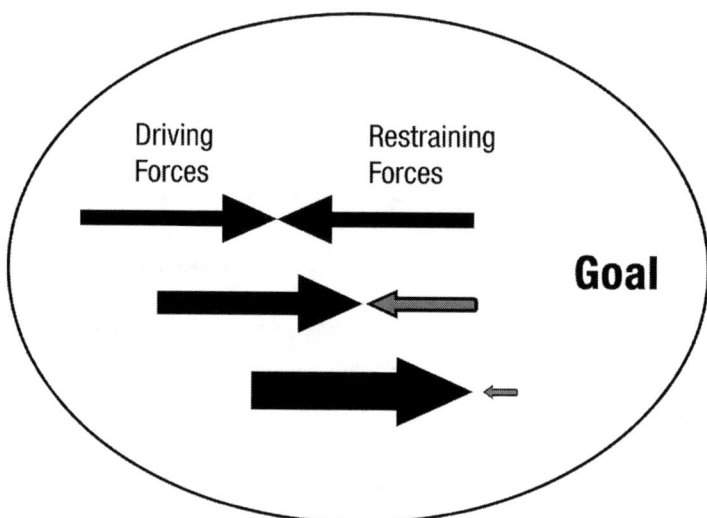

Weakening the restraining forces which releases the
driving forces in the direction of the goal.

Figure 8.8

A version of our force field adapted to work with teams and specific to each phase or subphase is illustrated in Figure 8.9. This prototypic force field guides our work with organizational work teams so that the interventions to the team are attuned to the context of the team's phase. Importantly, this force field formulates the phase conflicts in language congruent with an organizational context or consultation.

Systems-Centered Phases of Development in Work Groups

A Force Field of Driving and Restraining forces

Phase of Development	DRIVING FORCES →	← RESTRAINING FORCES
Authority Phase *Flight Subphase*	Developmental Goal: Create reality-testing culture →	← Implicit Goal: Don't rock the boat, play it safe
	Forming functional subgroups, asking "Anyone else?" →	← Maintaining social status communication, personalizing, stereotyped subgrouping
	Exploring →	← Explaining
	Specificity, bottom line →	← Vagueness, redundancy
	Data, reality-testing →	← Speculations
Fight Subphase	Developmental Goal: Explore differences in context of the work focus →	← Implicit Goal: Do it my way, repel invading differences
	Subgrouping around differences →	← "Yes, but" communications
	Recognizing and acknowledging frustrations →	← Complaining or blaming oneself, personalizing frustration
	Collecting data about hesitations →	← Blaming others, reacting to differences or withdrawing
	Making alternative proposals →	← Discharging in righteous outrage, indignation, sarcasm
Role Locks with Peers Subphase	Developmental Goal: Develop functional work role relationships with peers →	← Implicit Goal: Manage issues of dominance and control
	Clarifying work role relationships with peers →	← Creating one-up/down relationships
	Descriptive language →	← Personalizing language that induces role locks
Role Locks with Leader Subphase	Developmental Goal: Make a working relationship with one's leader and discover one's own authority →	← Implicit Goal: Sabotage authority, avoid responsibility, maintain status quo
	Clarifying differential role responsibilities →	← Complying or defying leader instead of task focus
	Learning to work with the leader one has →	← Making a case against the leader or organization
	Giving and taking authority →	← Blaming the leader, overtly or covertly
	Bring in what one knows & negotiate with leader →	← Denying one's own authority, or one's own competence
Collaboration Phase	Developmental Goal: Use differential resources of members while working in an interdependent team →	← Implicit Goal: Personal style at the expense of teamwork
	Contribute to positive work climate while exploring differences in the apparently similar →	← Focus on friendship at expense of work, never see differences to preserve affiliation
	Exploring similarities in the apparently different and work out a functional collaboration →	← Denial of similarities and insistence on working alone
	Take up team role →	← Go it alone or resist autonomy
Integration Phase	Developmental Goal: Work in role, goal & context →	← Implicit Goal: Self-focus at expense of system-focus, knowledge at expense of common sense or context
	Working in role & contributing to the goal & climate of the context →	← Blurring roles, ignoring goals & context, or only orienting to self-centered goals
	Using emotional and intellectual intelligence →	← Avoiding reality, resisting intuition or reasoning
	Common sense reality-testing →	← Losing common sense
	Maintaining a sense of humor →	← Losing perspective, personalizing
	Seeing the bigger picture →	← Self-focused at expense of context
	Using emotional knowledge in decision-making →	← Decisions without heart leading to ill-formed implementation
	Using the spirit of the law →	← Legalistic, letter of the law

Adapted from Y.M. Agazarian (1997) by Susan P. Gantt, SCT Conference, 2006.

Figure 8.9

Working within the phase context in psychotherapy groups

SCT discourages trying to weaken restraining forces that belong to later phases in early phase groups, as this premature work puts the system under stress by asking the system to do what it has not yet developed the resources to do. For example, there is often a strong push in new training or therapy groups in the flight sub-phase to work with intimacy. Since SCT emphasizes that how one talks is more related to the phase goal than what one talks about, the SCT leader continues to work to undo the flight restraining forces regardless of what the group talks about.

Claire: I am scared of being close and I want to have a close relationship.
Therapist: Are you scared right now?
C: Well, maybe I am.
T: Maybe? Does that mean you are scared, or you aren't? [Weakening the flight restraining force of ambiguity]
C: A little bit scared, yes.
T: Is that scare coming from something you are thinking, something you are feeling or from being at the edge of the unknown where everyone is apprehensive? [This question begins the work of undoing anxiety which is one of the restraining forces in the flight sub-phase, often from thoughts characterized by negative predictions] (Agazarian, 1997).

SCT sees each of the phases and subphases of system development as the context in which therapy takes place and, to reiterate, the context always determines what work can be done successfully. Doing only work that is phase-appropriate bypasses the frustrations and regressions that arise when work is attempted that patients or groups are not ready to do and instead sets up a potential win–win situation in which the patient or group succeeds step-by-step, each step paving the way for the next. When a group tries to explore intimacy before it has worked the earlier phases, flight restraining forces increase, as the group typically generates even more flight in explanations and speculations. Promoting premature change is iatrogenic and signals a lack of attunement to the context. Instead in SCT, by weakening phase-relevant restraining forces, the system then develops, establishes a new equilibrium, and learns to use its driving forces as resources for tackling the next set of phase-specific restraining forces. In other words, each phase builds the resources that function as a platform for the subsequent phase work. Using the SCT phases of system development as an orientation, SCT therapists, leaders and consultants weaken the restraining forces that are phase-relevant and congruent with the resources of the phase. This releases the resources of the phase-specific driving forces that support system development. Working with our phase model also led us to conceptualize each phase as a living human system that can be defined by its system variables.

Seeing SCT phases as living human systems

We have conceptualized each phase of system development as a living human system. Each phase and subphase can then be defined in terms of its goal, its boundary permeability (structure), its energy, and how it functions (what discriminations and integrations are possible). Each phase organizes energy with its boundary and discriminates and integrates this energy towards its specific goal of its phase of development.

For example, in the flight phase, though the energy/information will contain similarities and differences, the boundary opens much more to known similarities, as the implicit goal of flight is to avoid differences and not rock the boat. Thus, closing boundaries to differences and opening them to similarities meets the survival goal of maintaining flight. The phase will also be characterized by certain patterns of discrimination and integration, as some discriminations are possible in one phase yet not in another. For example, it is not too difficult to discriminate in the flight phase between experience in the here-and-now and experience generated by our thoughts about the future, negative or positive predictions.

In contrast, in the fight phase, if the group has not yet learned the difference between ambiguity and specificity, there is no resource for collecting data, and very little real work can be done to explore the frustration and irritation which arises in the fight phase. Establishing reality-testing is essential in all SCT work and vital in organizations and teams, for without the capacity to test reality (which is the developmental goal of the flight phase), decisions are made without real data and information is skewed in service of flight or fight. When a group does not do the developmental work in the flight phase of learning to be specific, then there is no capacity to explore rather than enact in the fight phase. This is a good example of how each phase lays the foundation for the work of the later phase.

Integrating the role-systems map with phases of system development

With the addition of the role-systems map, each phase can now be defined as a hierarchy of isomorphic systems containing inner-person, inter-person, and whole system roles. For example, the flight subphase will be defined by its inner-person roles (e.g., prototypic flight phase secondary survivor roles are the identified patient and helper), its inter-person roles either functionally subgrouping to explore the phase conflicts or enacting the helper/identified patient role lock, and its whole system roles with its implicit goal of fixating in flight and its explicit goal of establishing norms that help the group function.

Recognizing the system-as-a-whole role-system is more challenging. On the one hand, the roles that are elicited by system-as-a-whole dynamics look just like all the other roles that represent the inner-person or inter-person systems. It is only when one recognizes that there are specific sets of roles that identify the flight phase of development which are different from all the other predicted sets of roles that identify the other different phases that we can discover the role inductions of the system-as-a-whole and in turn its implicit goal and role.

Being able to intuit the implicit influence of the system-as-a-whole that elicits our role-system responses allows us to see the influence of the phase context. It is more familiar to most of us to see what it is in the context of our personal experience that elicits our inner-person and inter-person role responses. Seeing the system-as-a-whole influence requires us to observe ourselves when we are induced and develop awareness of our own characteristic role locks in our responses to the identified patient in the flight phase, to the scapegoat in the fight phase, to sadistic or masochistic impulses in the crisis of hatred, and to merging or alienating in the intimacy phase. Awareness of the context of the system-as-a-whole can be as complex as a phase of development in a person, a group, an organization or a nation on many dimensions. For example, a person, group or nation with many available resources will serve as a different context from ones that are not resourceful. Contexts are systems characterized by a specific phase that influence and maintain the role-systems that they generate. It is important for us not to overlook that we are talking about the phase as part of the context when we remind ourselves of "role, goal and context."

The whole system context is defined by its phase with its phase norms which are operationally defined by its force field of driving and restraining forces. As a goal-directing system, each phase will have a developmental goal linked to its driving forces (D-goal for short in Figure 8.10) and a competing implicit goal implied by its restraining forces (survival goal or S-goal for short). The survivor goal will always be oriented to the survival of the phase as it is, "the phase as it is" is the "known," which contrasts with developing into a new phase, the "unknown."

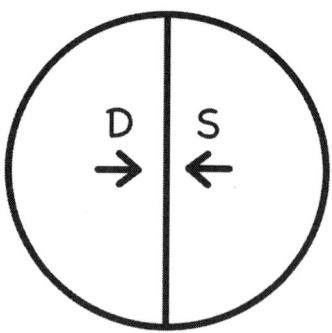

Figure 8.10

For example, in the flight subphase the survival goal is to avoid any differences – this survival goal is implied by the restraining forces in flight whereas the driving forces imply the developmental goal. Since the role-system hierarchy for each phase is isomorphic, these restraining forces and their implicit survivor goal will be reiterated at each system level, in the inner, inter and whole system levels.

Summary

We have recounted some of the influences on our phase model that seeded and supported our work as we were integrating our systems theory and formulating and operationally defining our phases of system development. Integrating our work from SAVI enabled us to see phases as whole system communication patterns whose approach and avoidance communications could then be linked to a force field of driving and restraining forces. This led us to formulate a force field to operationally define each developmental phase and subphase and, in revisiting our theory, to conceptualize each phase as a living human system that can be defined as a hierarchy of isomorphic role-systems, each of which can be operationally defined as a force of driving and restraining vectors.

In our next chapter, we elaborate both our overall force field guide and the implications of seeing phases as a hierarchy of isomorphic role-systems. We conclude with discussing the implications of both for how SCT works with phases, phase dynamics and phase development in the context of whole system communication patterns.

References

Agazarian, Y. M. (1968). *A theory of verbal behaviour and information transfer*. Temple University. Retrieved from UMI Dissertation Express. (AAT 6914069)

Agazarian, Y. M. (1997). *Systems-centered therapy for groups*. New York, NY: Guilford Press. Reprinted in paperback (2004). London, UK: Karnac Books.

Agazarian, Y. M. (2003). Book review. [Review of the book *Traumatic experience in the unconscious life of groups*, by E. Hopper]. *Systems-Centered News*, 11(1), 3–4.

Agazarian, Y. M. (2012). Preface. In R. Lenn & K. Stefano (Eds.), *Small, large and median groups: The work of Patrick de Maré* (pp. xix–xxiv). London, UK: Karnac Books.

Agazarian, Y. M., & Gantt, S. P. (2000). *Autobiography of a theory: Developing a theory of living human systems and its systems-centered practice*. London, UK: Jessica Kingsley.

Bennis, W. G., & Shepard, H. A. (1956). A theory of group development. *Human Relations*, 9(4), 415–437. doi:10.1177/001872675600900403

Bion, W. R. (1961). *Experiences in groups*. London, UK: Tavistock.

Bion, W. R. (1963). *Elements of psycho-analysis*. London, UK: William Heinemann. Reprinted (1984). London, UK: Karnac Books.

Bridger, H. (1987). Courses and working conferences as transitional learning institutions. In W. Brendan Reddy & C. C. Henderson (Eds.), *Training, theory and practice*. Washington, DC: NTL Institute/University Associates.

Bridger, H. (1990). The discovery of the therapeutic community: The Northfield experiments. In E. Trist, H. Murray, & B. Trist (Eds.), *The social engagement of social science: A*

Tavistock anthology: Vol. I: The socio-psychological perspective (pp. 68–87). Baltimore, MD: University of Pennsylvania Press.

Festinger, L. (1953). Informal social communication. In D. Cartwright & A. Zander (Eds.), *Group dynamics, research and theory*. Evanston, IL: Row, Peterson.

Gantt, S. P., & Agazarian, Y. M. (2007). Phases of system development in organizational work groups: The systems-centered approach for intervening in context. *Organisational & Social Dynamics, 7*(2), 253–291.

Hopper, E. (2003). *Traumatic experience in the unconscious life of groups*. London, UK: Jessica Kingsley.

Lenn, R., & Stefano, K. (Eds.). (2012). *Small, large and median groups: The work of Patrick de Maré*. London, UK: Karnac Books.

Lewin, K. (1951). *Field theory in social science*. New York, NY: Harper & Row.

Shannon, C. E., & Weaver, W. (1964). *The mathematical theory of communication*. Urbana, IL: University of Illinois Press.

Simon, A., & Agazarian, Y. M. (1967). *SAVI: Sequential analysis of verbal interaction*. Philadelphia, PA: Research for Better Schools.

Simon, A., & Agazarian, Y. M. (2000). SAVI: The system for analyzing verbal interaction. In A. Beck & C. Lewis (Eds.), *The process of group psychotherapy: Systems for analyzing change* (pp. 357–380). Washington, DC: American Psychological Association.

Chapter 9

Putting the phases of system development into practice

We are not alone in using the idea of phases of group development. The idea of phases or stages in group development is widespread in the group literature, with over 2,500 articles listed in a recent search through EBSCO PsycINFO.[1] Yet in spite of this popularity, phases in group development are not universally acknowledged in the group field, for example, neither Tavistock nor group analysis use group phase models per se. Of the various phase models, the earliest and still most influential article on phases of group development, both for SCT and the group field in general, is that of Bennis and Shepard (1956), whose contributions we discussed in our last chapter.

Brabender and Fallon (2009) have provided a comprehensive review of the history of group phase models. They emphasize the usefulness of a developmental focus for enabling patients to see how their experience is related to their context. This is especially important in SCT, where seeing the context is an alternative to personalizing. Brabender and Fallon also emphasize that a group developmental framework makes it easier to see the various levels of the group, the individual, dyads, subgroups and the group-as-a-whole and gives a context for what might be usefully processed in group interventions across theoretical frameworks. Most importantly, they emphasized that "group psychotherapy is a more effective treatment when the therapist considers group developmental issues" (p. 3).

Why group phase matters in SCT

SCT sees the system phase as an essential part of the context and, as we have emphasized, the phase determines what work a group can do and cannot do. For example, in the flight phase, a group or team avoids differences. In contrast, in the fight phase, members actively scan for differences and attempt to convert them or easily move to scapegoating them. In neither phase does the group easily integrate differences. This is quite significant for us, as SCT sees the discrimination and integration of differences as the heart of the process by which all living human systems survive, develop and transform. This has led us to emphasize how to work with the phase dynamics in each phase in a way that differences, so essential for development and transformation, can be integrated.

SCT's phases of system development

SCT has identified three phases of system development: authority, intimacy and work.

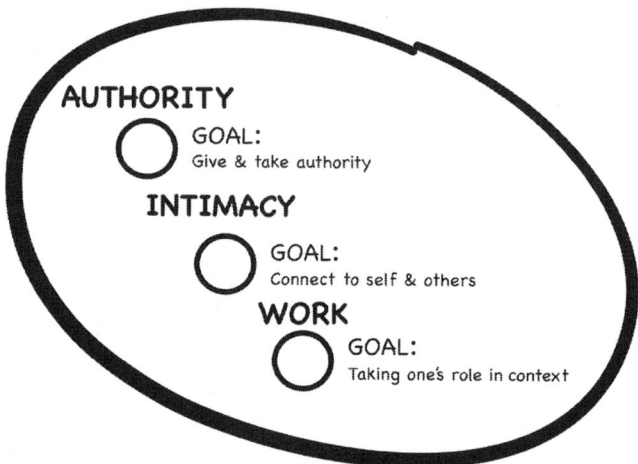

PHASES OF SYSTEM DEVELOPMENT

AUTHORITY

GOAL:
Give & take authority

INTIMACY

GOAL:
Connect to self & others

WORK

GOAL:
Taking one's role in context

Figure 9.1

We have then defined each phase in terms of its developmental goal (see Figure 9.1). In the authority phase, the developmental goal is to give and take authority. In the intimacy phase, the goal is to intimately connect to oneself and others. In the phase of interdependent work, love and play, the goal is to take up one's role, goal and context with all that one knows.

Summary of the phases of system development

SCT divides the three overall phases of system development (authority, intimacy and work) into subphases. We have operationally defined each phase or subphase as a predictable set of driving and restraining forces (Agazarian, 1986; Agazarian & Gantt, 2000, 2003; Gantt & Agazarian, 2007). SCT systematically weakens the phase-relevant restraining forces so that the driving forces are released towards the developmental goal of the phase or subphase. Releasing driving forces changes the system's equilibrium, develops the system and creates a more sustainable path for ongoing system development. When the developmental goal is met, the system transforms into the next phase, with its specific goal and predictable force field.

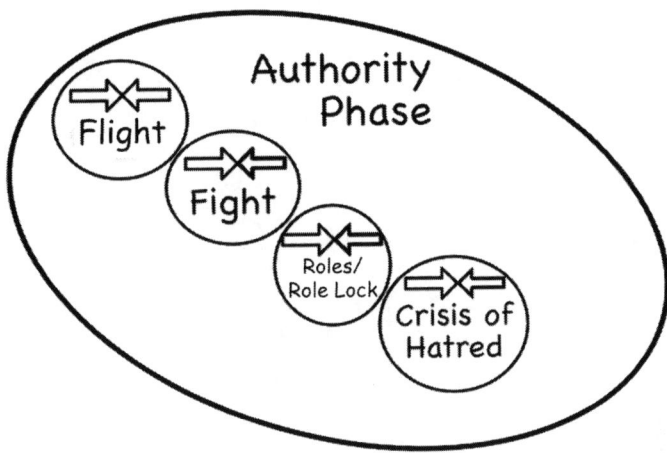

Figure 9.2

First phase of system development: relationship to authority

The authority phase, the first phase of system development, is divided into four subphases (see Figure 9.2): flight, the transition to fight, roles and role locks, and the crisis of hatred (which is fueled by the negative transference). Each subphase is then operationally defined by the force field prototypic to the phase.

The authority phase is oriented around one's relationships to society, to one's own authority and to others' authority. In therapy, this reflects the reality that people enter therapy as already socialized human beings who have learned to relate to their life in the world in both adaptive and maladaptive ways. In the process of becoming socialized, people learn to adapt the way they think and speak, the way they behave, and the way they feel. This phase is especially important in working in organizations that are primarily fixated in the authority phase over issues of power and control.

Working in the authority phase in therapy and training

In this first subphase in therapy, SCT works to restore the patients' natural connection to their mind and reality-testing (flight subphase), to the body and emotions (transition to fight subphase), and to one's centering self to regain fuller access to both verbal and emotional intelligence, in the service of giving and taking authority. This is done by systematically reducing the restraining forces or defenses that interfere or constrict people's access to their self-knowledge. This frees the driving forces to move the system towards its developmental goals (see Figure 9.3).

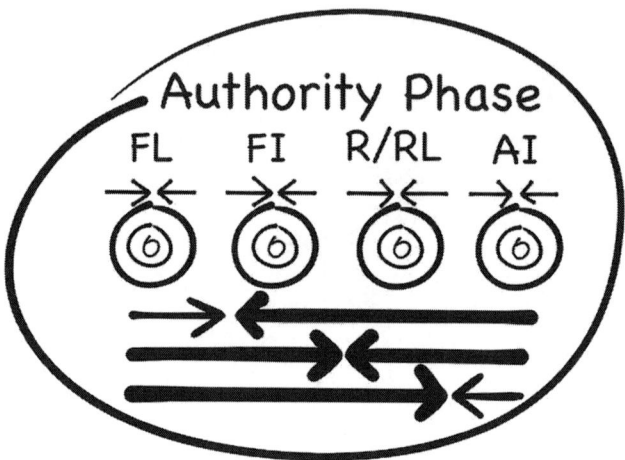

Figure 9.3

Early in the subphase of flight (see Figure 9.4), SCT modifies the restraining force of anxiety. For example, the group learns to undo the negative predictions that generate anxiety. This is done almost immediately to preempt the group from using these defenses we all use in everyday life to manage our anxiety. Also, in flight, SCT interrupts the tendency of all groups to move into social behavior by importing and establishing outside social norms in the group and instead establishes the norm of functional subgrouping.

FLIGHT from the present and from differences	
Exploring →	← Explaining
Learning to subgroup by saying "anybody else" at the end of message (systems-centered) →	← Personalizing communications & remaining self-centered
Clear & specific communications →	← Vague, ambiguous communications
Exploring wish to be given care →	← Creating an identified patient role
Giving care in response to genuine care-seeking →	← Creating a care-taking/helper role
Reality-testing, undoing anxiety-provoking thoughts →	← Negative predictions & mindreads
Discriminating between tension & the experience contained within the tension →	← Tension
Discriminating how present is different from the past →	← Relating to present "as if" it is the past

Figure 9.4

In the transition subphase from flight to fight (see Figure 9.5), the depressive subgroup learns to recognize that turning their retaliatory impulse against themselves results in depression (see Figure 9.6), whereas turning it out allows the group to decondition its fear of anger and learn not to take each other's aggression just personally. SCT understands aggression as energy for managing frustrations, while outrage and tantrums are a defense against the life force energy that aggression contains.

Transition to FIGHT over differences		
Exploring →	←	Enacting
Subgrouping around differences →	←	Saying yes, but; monologues disguised as a dialogue
Joining the "deviant" & exploring similarities →	←	Scapegoating differences
Undoing the boomerang of depression & exploring the retaliatory impulse →	←	Discharging against the self by turning retaliatory impulse back on the self in depression
Recognizing outrage as different from anger, and centering to discover the feeling →	←	Discharging in outrage
Exploring & containing irritability, aggression & life force →	←	Hostile acting out of frustration, irritability, aggression & life force

Figure 9.5

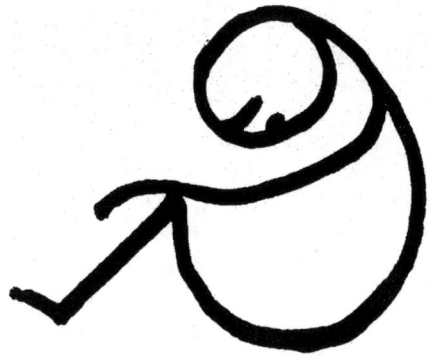

Figure 9.6

In the subphase of roles and role locks, members learn how to observe how person-centered roles from the past induce others to retreat into reciprocal personal roles (see Figures 9.7 and 9.8) that fixate the group and distract from the group's working in the present.

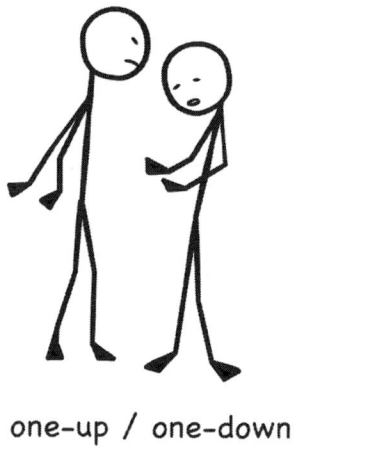 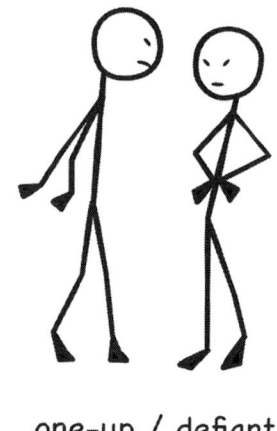

one-up / one-down   one-up / defiant

Figure 9.7

ROLES AND ROLE LOCKS with each other	
Naming the role & the experience in the → role, identifying its here-and-now trigger & the outputs from the role that induce others	← Repeating old interpersonal roles, creating & enacting one-up & one-down role relationship; identified patient & helper; scapegoater & scapegoat; defiant & compliant or dominant & submissive
Exploring role triggers & role inductions →	← Enacting role induction & role suction
Recognizing role as past adaptation to a → past context	← Living in past "as if" present

Figure 9.8

By learning to give and receive descriptive and impersonal feedback, the group members weaken the inevitable role locks that easily surface for people where there is a good match for their repetition compulsion. Experiencing the freedom from old roles frees the energy in aggression (very different from hostility). This typically develops a good supportive climate among members as they learn from each other. This then makes a foundation for members to explore their underlying conviction that the only problem with the group is the leader. Exploring this conviction marks the transition from the subphase of roles/role locks into the crisis of hatred.

The work in each of the subphases contributes resources and builds skills that develop the group and its capacity to work through the crisis of hatred (see Figure 9.9). By exploring hatred of the authority and reclaiming the energy of hatred, rather than constricting it in roles in relation to others' authority and authority with oneself, the group works through their authority issues. The group and its members then discover their own authority and gain freedom from blaming and externalizing.

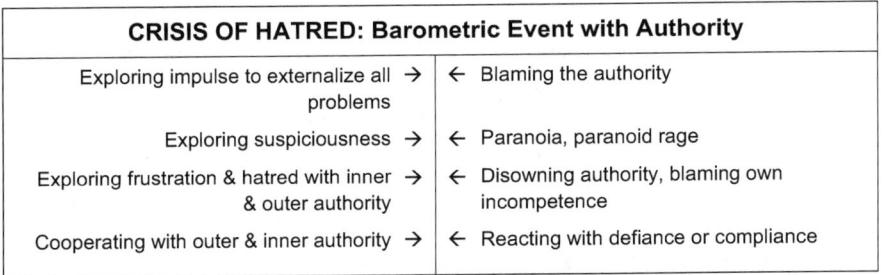

CRISIS OF HATRED: Barometric Event with Authority	
Exploring impulse to externalize all → problems	← Blaming the authority
Exploring suspiciousness →	← Paranoia, paranoid rage
Exploring frustration & hatred with inner → & outer authority	← Disowning authority, blaming own incompetence
Cooperating with outer & inner authority →	← Reacting with defiance or compliance

Figure 9.9

In newer groups, the authority issue can be fun. For example, in one workshop, this work started when one member looked at me (Yvonne) and said, "you are no spring chicken." The group enthusiastically joined him and, in no time at all, developed their fantasy. They fantasized putting me in a pot with carrots and celery, putting the pot on a fire, and dancing around the fire with great glee, chanting a cooking song. There was a big release of energy, and the group made the transition into the intimacy phase with a lot of energy for work.

As many therapists and group leaders know, the crisis of hatred is based on deep social dynamics, and the ability to explore these dynamics requires group development over time. Group after group will reinvent the killing and eating of the leader to give them strength and establish their survival. And as many therapists know – it is very important (though sometimes almost impossible) not to take a group's crisis of hatred just personally! The crisis of hatred is the fulcrum event that allows the group to transition into the phase of intimacy. It is important for SCT leaders to learn to interrupt and deflect any tendency for the group to become fixated in a gratifying intimacy before the energy in aggression and the de-idealizations have taken place. Enchantment is very gratifying, but not at the cost of maturity.

Working in the authority phase in organizations and with teams

In organizations, the goal in the authority phase is to learn to give and take authority in one's role to support the goal of one's context (Agazarian & Philibossian, 1998; Gantt, 2013; Gantt & Agazarian, 2007). The work establishes reality-testing by weakening flight into ambiguity, opens access to the energy of frustration to use the energy for work, and enables shifts out of members' past adaptive roles and role locks like one-up and one-down, or dominant and submissive, that prevent them from taking their work roles with peers and authorities (see Figure 8.9). Ultimately, members and teams learn to work with the leader they have, who is always different from the leader they want, and to enable their leader to succeed. In turn, members learn to take their own authority to lead in context and in their roles. Undoing the restraining forces releases the driving forces for development and consequently greater productivity. Importantly, across industry groups, Wheelan, whose phase model was also derivative from Bennis and Shepard (1956), found that work groups with more development evidenced greater productivity and those with less development, lower productivity (Wheelan, Burchill, & Tilin, 2003; Wheelan & Kesselring, 2005; Wheelan & Lisk, 2000; Wheelan, Murphy, Tsumura, & Fried Kline, 1998; Wheelan & Tilin, 1999).

Second phase of development: intimacy

The work in the intimacy phase is with the driving and restraining forces to separation/individuation. Observing one's subgrouping style is often useful for members in identifying their own challenges in the process of separation/individuation. For example, members who tend to join every subgroup that comes along also tend to have difficulty separating, while those members for whom no subgroup is quite right tend to have difficulty individuating. The intimacy phase work builds upon the insights into projective identification that occurred, at a greater or lesser depth, in exploring the dynamics of the repetition compulsion dynamics that are worked initially in the authority phase. Thinking isomorphy, these same authority dynamics have underpinnings in the intimacy phase just as the social roles are related to the affiliative/attachment roles.

Having undone the pull to externalize difficulties and blame authority, others' and our own authority, work with intimacy leads to the recognition that one cannot relate to another until one can first relate to oneself. In this second phase, the focus changes from a preoccupation with authority to how to make relationships with oneself *and* others. It is then that people come to understand that one can never have the relationship one wants; one can only have the relationship one can make! The relationships one can make, of course, require coming out of the fantasy of the perfect relationship and into the reality that every relationship is a compromise. Learning to live in a world where we can bear and accept the differences in the other is never our favorite thing, yet it is how we and the systems in which we have member-ship develop.

Working with intimacy conflicts in therapy and training

The SCT approach to our defenses against intimacy is both simpler and more profound than work with the defenses in the authority phase. The dynamics are profound in that they have roots in the basic good–bad split, a primary dis-crimination made by all of us before we have developed the ability to integrate. This pre-integration level is always available in all of us (often at the level of our affiliative/attachment roles), and we regress to this split under sufficiently stressful conditions. On the good side, all is right with the world as long as we experience a mirroring and attuned relationship. On the bad side, nothing is ever good enough and we reject mirroring, attunement and empathy.

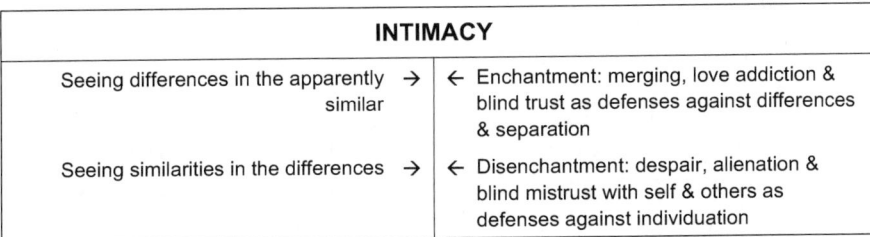

INTIMACY	
Seeing differences in the apparently → similar	← Enchantment: merging, love addiction & blind trust as defenses against differences & separation
Seeing similarities in the differences →	← Disenchantment: despair, alienation & blind mistrust with self & others as defenses against individuation

Figure 9.10

Intimacy is also the phase in which SCT therapists have more in common with psychodynamic therapists in our work with the separation/individua-tion dynamics than in the first phase where SCT leaders actively intervene to set SCT norms. Dependency dynamics are explored in this phase (see Fig-ure 9.10), both as they relate to the dependency impulses to be as one with others in enchanted blind trust (the good side of the split) and as they relate to the counter-dependent impulses to be distant from others in disenchantment and blind mistrust (the bad side of the split). These phase dynamics fuel, and are fueled by, our affiliative/attachment role-systems.

The basic SCT methods for explicitly recognizing differences in the appar-ently similar and similarities in the apparently different are essential in this phase. Recognizing differences in what is apparently similar between oneself and others enables us to separate. Recognizing similarities in what is apparently different between oneself and others enables us to individuate without fear that we will lose our identity in relationships.

Also in this phase, SCT has pioneered how to work with the prototypic intimacy conflicts by having the group containing and exploring the two prototypic role-systems (enchanted role and disenchanted role) in parallel subgroups, with first one subgroup exploring and then the other. In this way of working, the whole system contains the two subgroups simultaneously and is able at some point to integrate the similarities in what is apparently different. Listening to the group work as the enchanted subgroup explores sounds like a harmonious flow:

> "I love this group." "It is the best." "Couldn't be better." "Wish we could be here always, this is how life should be. Maybe we could stay together forever." "Yes, just like we are, no one else, maybe live on an island together." "Oh yes, that sounds wonderful."

At some point the difference comes in: "That feels a little much to me" and the disenchanted subgroup explores:

> "Yes, I agree, nothing about that sounds real." "Can't really count on anyone, better to stay alone." "Never felt connected. Connection is not really real. I don't even connect to myself."

As this work continues, those in the disenchanted subgroup start to recognize the similarities in what was initially different. They start to feel close to each other and to enjoy feeling understood and together with others who also feel disenchanted. In turn, the enchanted subgroup begins to notice differences in what was apparently similar, for example, discovering that "forever" feels like a bit much and maybe boring.

These SCT methods for managing the dynamics of intimacy are highly containing, and still the two most challenging experiences to explore in the phases of intimacy are the experience of emptiness and the fear of falling apart. SCT reframes these experiences so that patients and trainees can explore these with the natural apprehension about going into the unknown, rather than believing them to be dangerous or pathological.

Working with collaboration issues in organizations and teams

The conflicts in intimacy fuel the collaboration conflicts that dominate work groups and teams in organizations as they learn to collaborate with differential resources. The developmental work in this phase of a team is to learn to collaborate on structure, function and goal orientation and weaken any of the restraining forces to this collaboration. SCT works differently in the work context than in training or therapy, as the relevant work is related to work collaboration though the conflicts are still fueled by the underlying dynamics related to intimacy. In all of this work, the focus is linked to goal achievement in the work context.

Issues of affiliation and friendship for some clash with the issues of others who prefer working alone. Those leaning towards affiliation (Schutz, 1958) find it difficult to disagree with those they like, resulting in a focus on climate at the expense of task. Those who like working alone emphasize their differences at the cost of noticing similarities, and of inclusion, and may tend to focus on task at the expense of building a collaborative climate.

(Gantt & Agazarian, 2007, p. 280)

Work phase

The ongoing task of the mature group is to enable communications across the boundaries at every level: personal boundaries, member boundaries, subgroup boundaries, and boundaries of the group-as-a-whole. In the ongoing facts of group life, in and out of therapy, the conflicts inherent to the process of communication do not change, nor do the problems that lie on the path to the goals, but the ability to work with them does change.

(Agazarian, 1999, p. 104)

We could also say that the work in this phase in both therapy and organizations is the ongoing work of learning to know what one knows apprehensively and comprehensively and to use this knowing in one's role related to the goal of the context (see Figure 9.11). In organizations the ongoing work in every organization and team is to learn to see one's role, moment to moment, and to take one's role in context. SCT's model of role, goal and context (Gantt, 2005, 2013; Gantt & Agazarian, 2004, 2005, 2007; Solomon-Gillis & Trey, 1997) is the heart of ongoing development in the organizational context.

Overall, the phases of development follow a specific sequence, which does not mean that groups do not briefly experience phases out of sequence. In fact, these deviations actually allow members of one-day or two-day workshops to have a taste of all the phases. For example, in a one-day workshop in England,

WORK & PLAY	
Putting one's heart into work, play & → relationships	← Working & playing without commitment
Using common sense to implement the → spirit	← Following the letter of the law & not the spirit
Using common sense in relationship to → the larger picture	← Seeing *only* the details & failing to recognize the larger picture
Using both one's apprehensive & → comprehensive information for solving problems (emotional intelligence)	← Following *only* one's comprehension or *only* one's apprehensive intuition for solving problems

Figure 9.11

the group had a good experience in the work phase. Before lunch, one sub-group was concerned that they did not understand how one could free oneself from lifetime patterns of behavior that kept them in their old roles. A different subgroup could not see how they would ever understand the group-as-a-whole as a system. After lunch, the group surfaced a fantasy of being different animals coming together around a watering hole. As the fantasy built, members explored more deeply the experience of being the animal each had become. As the "animal members" fantasized about all being together around the watering hole, there was an astonishing moment when a member (who had not been able to join the fantasy) exclaimed: "Oh my goodness, my hand has become a paw! No, really, I mean it, but I don't know what animal it belongs to! Oh! Oh yes, I do. I'm a bear!" She became solid in her chair and looked just like a bear. Earlier, she had been working on an old role in which she took so much responsibility for groups that she could hardly "bear" it. Then she said "I'm not at this watering hole all alone! My bear is not the only one who is responsible. I've got a subgroup!" "Me too," said another member. He had been recognizing his timidity and fear of speaking up in the group, using a very soft voice and looking very small in his chair. But at the watering hole, he was fully in his chair – he looked big and had a presence that could not be discounted. "Oh my god," he said. "I'm a lion! I'm a lion and I have a roar . . . I have a big roar inside me. I'm here. I'm to be reckoned with." We all believed him. Then a third member spoke up. She had been unable to get the concept of the group as a system, simply could not see it. She was a tall, thin woman, and often looked as if she sat in a way to make herself look smaller. But now she was sitting tall and looking around the group with great interest. "I'm a giraffe," she announced. "I can see you all around the watering hole – and we *are* a system!"

Integrating our phases of system development and our role-systems map

Our earlier work in Chapter 8 laid the foundation for integrating these two maps: the force field map of our phases of system development and our role-systems map. First, the phase of development is an essential part of each of the nested system contexts in our role-system hierarchy: inner-person, inter-person or whole system.

Using isomorphy, we can infer that the phase of any one of these nested systems will reflect and influence the phase in each of these isomorphic systems in our role-system hierarchy (see Figure 9.12). The isomorphy changes as the system context changes. The same phase will manifest differently in the context of each system level. In addition, each phase is also itself a different context. The role activation will be different in the inner-person system dependent on the whole system phase context and its phase conflicts, which are different in different phases. Put another way, the phase of the whole system functions as the supra-system in relation to the inter-person system which is the containing system for the inner-person system and as such will influence both up and down

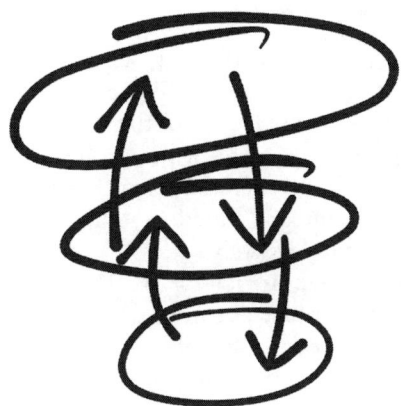

Figure 9.12

the hierarchy. In turn, both the inter- and inner-person system's outputs will be elicited by the phase and contribute to and influence the phase of development. Thus, working with any system level will affect the other system levels. Further, we can identify that weakening the phase-relevant restraining forces in the inter-person, the middle level system, will be the most influential change strategy.

Each phase of system development has identifiable triggers that stimulate survivor roles related to the phase dynamics. Each phase is also then recognizable by its predictable survivor roles stimulated by the specific phase conflicts which function to keep the system stable and in the known. Staying in the known stability of the phase is an implicit (survival) goal in each phase. The alternative role-system is inter-person interdependence with centered awareness of role, goal and context; for example, in a training group, the role is subgrouping to explore the phase conflicts.

To recap, the whole system context will embody the phase dynamics that are operative and will be identifiable by its force field of driving and restraining forces at all system levels. Systems-centered groups use functional subgrouping to explore the dynamics and conflicts that the whole system phase-norms embody. The whole system also contains group-specific norms, which can be driving or restraining depending on the goal. For example, the essential norm in an SCT group is functional subgrouping which requires inter-person expression and exploration whereas, in contrast, the norms in a psychodynamic group are more oriented to inner-person expression and exploration. In SCT, inner-person conflicts are explored in inter-person subgrouping with others who resonate as a subgroup voice for the group and often another subgroup which contains and explores the other side of the conflict. From our view, the phases and phase conflicts in an SCT group are similar to the phases in a psychodynamic group, yet the norms of each group are very different so that the work in each phase will look and progress differently.

Attuning to the phase context: the work in each phase through our role-systems map

Integrating the role-systems map with our phase model has enabled us to resonate with the whole system level more easily and hear and see the role-system outputs at all system levels as expressions of the phase context. We can say that the role-system outputs are the voice of the group's phase. From this way of seeing, one can infer the group system's implicit goals which will, thinking isomorphy, be similar in structure and function at all levels of the system – inner-person, inter-person and whole system.

Attuning to the phase context is vital for SCT leaders. In fact, in SCT, working without awareness of the phase dynamics as the context for the work signals a survival goal, closed to awareness of role, goal and context. Phase dynamics contain the implicit, survival system goal. In SCT, recognizing and addressing the implicit goal is fundamental, as weakening the restraining forces that maintain the implicit goal frees driving forces for the primary goal of every living human system which is to survive, develop and transform. Role-system outputs are important data for recognizing the implicit system goal.

Examples of role-system outputs in the flight subphases

Role-systems in the authority subphases are social role-systems. Our social roles originated in our various role adaptations when being socialized with authorities in our early life. These social role-systems develop at the boundary between our inner-person system where our primary goal is "me" and our inter-person system which is all about "we." Our social roles are triggered by the context of the authority subphases and their implicit goals and, in turn, outputs from these social roles enable us to identify the implicit goals.

For example, in the flight subphase, the implicit goals are to stay safe, not rock the boat, take no chances, and avoid the present. The social survival roles activated in this context are roles like identified patient, helper, explainer. These closed boundaried role-systems protected and maintained our essential relationships with our socializing figures, for example, parents, teachers, coaches. In the present, these adaptations relate to the past (and often induce role locks in the present). What is more, they are at the expense of our present inter-person goals of solving the problem of how to take membership in the here-and-now in a new group and context. When these role-system outputs into the inter-person system induce reciprocal roles and role locks in the group context, they will maintain flight, stereotyping and social status communications at the expense of reality-testing and inter-person data collection in the here-and-now. In modifying these role-system outputs, SCT leaders are activating an explorer role in the inner-person *and* changing the role-system output, both of which help the role-system itself develop.

Revisiting the force field in the flight subphase (refer again to Figure 9.4), a common intervention would be to point out vagueness and ask for specificity

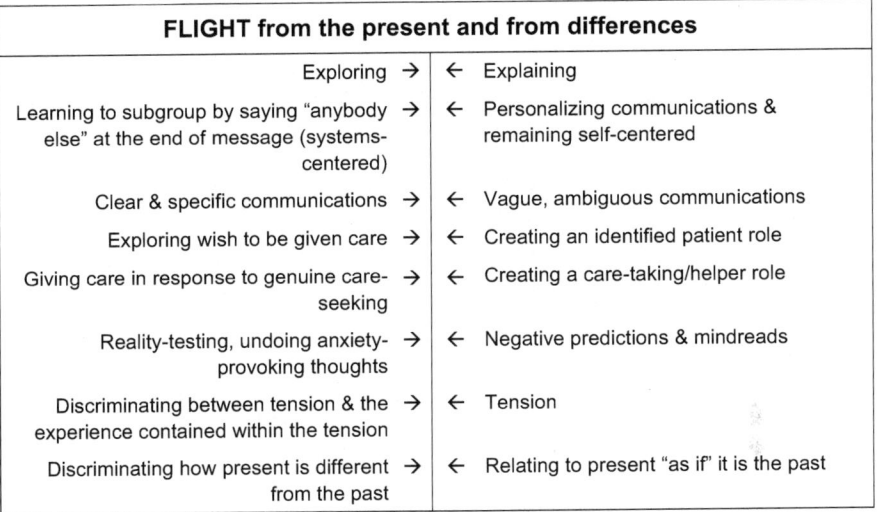

Figure 9.4

to weaken a flight restraining force. This kind of intervention is an input to the survival role-system which can be a step in developing the role-system. For example, a group member saying "I might be sad or maybe I am just tired; it's hard to really know how I feel" is likely to induce some others in the group into a care-taking or helper role, which could easily become an identified patient/care-taker role lock for the group-as-a-whole. By pointing out the vagueness and asking the member to experiment with being specific instead, the member can find out if being specific helps them get understood. In this way, the leader reorients the member to the communication goal and role rather than the survivor goal and role. This boundarying intervention reduces the noise in the communication output, interrupts the incipient role lock in the group and also vectors the member towards his or her inter-person system role where the goal is communication to others.

Though our theoretical work with role-systems is relatively new, we have worked for many years with modifying noise in communication in the flight phase system. This builds valid communication, establishes functional sub-grouping and creates a reality-testing culture which not only weakens the flight restraining forces but also develops resources for working in the present. More recently, based on our hypothesis that came out of rethinking vectors, as we discussed in Chapter 4, we have been observing how modifying the role-system output not only weakens the restraining force in the phase and builds valid communication but also functions to develop the survivor role-system itself. This has led us to begin experimenting with how to introduce the role-systems map itself as a tool to help ourselves, our clients and our groups work with the challenges of each phase. Next we describe an example of doing this in the flight phase of development.

Introducing the role-systems map to our groups in the flight subphase

We start by introducing the idea that recognizing our behavior and language can enable us to identify our role-system. Once we know our role-system, we can identify how our role-system is fueled by our inner-person system (survivor or explorer), our inter-person system (role lock) or our whole system (phase). We can then use our map in Figure 9.13 to let us explore how to travel around in ourselves from different role-systems in our different person systems.

Here are the questions we can ask (see Figure 9.14) ourselves or others to help map our role-systems in the flight subphase:

Role-Systems Map

life force energy
Survivor →
exploratory drive
Explorer

exploratory
energy →
development

organizing
energy →
transformation

Inner-Person

E ←→ S

present   past
adaptive   adaptive
roles   roles

subgroups   role induction
at all   role locks
levels

Inter-Person

System Hierarchy

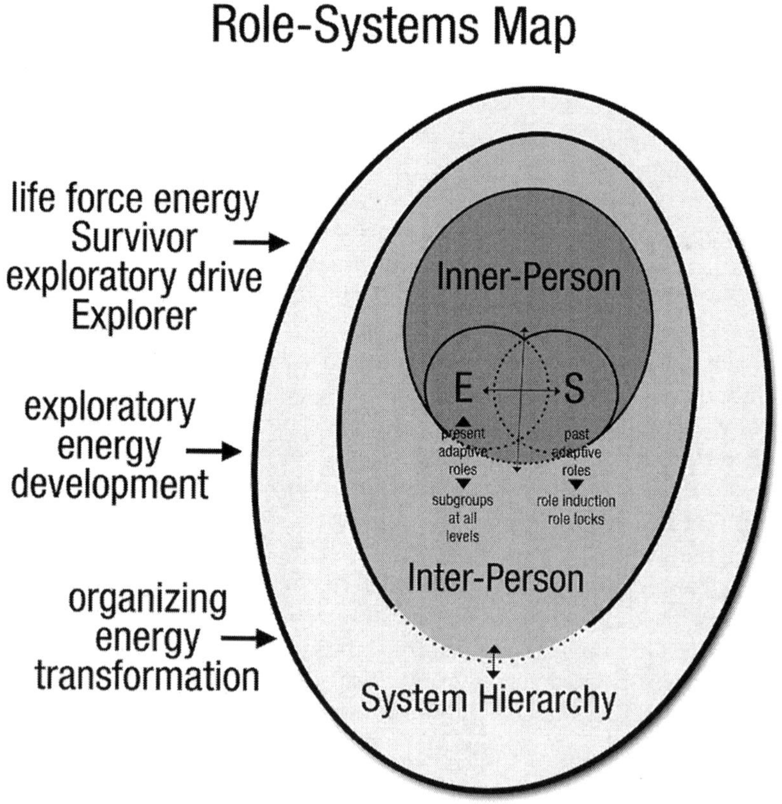

Figure 9.13

FLIGHT SUBPHASE

INNER-PERSON ROLE-SYSTEMS

Am I in my inner-person self, taking things personally, anxious or tense perhaps, or remembering look-alikes from the past?

Or am I in my curious self, open to myself with curiosity about myself?

Personal Present Curious Survivor Role-System:

Am I personalizing my experience, shutting out others but open to myself and curious about my own experience?

If yes, then I am in what SCT calls my curious survivor role-system.

Personal Past Closed Survivor Role-System:

Am I personalizing my experience and out of touch with myself, or scaring myself with look-alikes in my past, where I re-experience being anxious and tense and unsure how to behave, with impulses to hide and be "good" like I was then?

Or maybe the opposite, did I overcome my fear and leap into the fray?

Am I experiencing the present "as if" it is the past?

If yes, then we know we have retreated into old survivor role-systems that we developed to adapt when we felt insecure and alone, maybe hoping for someone to make it better or maybe we adapted by trying to fix it for others.

If we become curious and recognize that our behavior is familiar to us, we can use this map and identify which system we are living in, and decide which system we would rather be in, and get curious about how to change both our system context and our role.

INTER-PERSON ROLE-SYSTEMS

Are we noticing when our focus shifts from just our internal experience or, on the map, have we changed into our inter-person self with a role-system that lets us become aware of our relationship to both ourselves and others as well as the goals outside ourselves with others and in the context?

Importantly, have we crossed the boundary into the inter-person system by importing our past survivor systems like "helper" or "fixer" or "take charge" or "not knowing what to do" or "hiding" or "being good" or "jumping in," all important past adaptations stimulated by the flight phase dynamics?

Or are we in a present inter-person system that we are developing in ourselves with others in the context of the here-and-now present?

Figure 9.14

These questions have been useful to us as well as our trainees and patients. They like using the person-as-a-system illustration as well and it seems to make it easier to see oneself objectively when looking at the picture to explore and observe. A longtime group member a few weeks after the group had been using the illustration brought in how he was starting to be curious whether he was importing the survivor role he learned with his father of never being good enough with his wife.

Predictable social survival roles in each phase

Each of the authority subphases will have predictable social role-systems that are activated, triggered by the subphase, its dynamics and conflicts, as summarized in Figure 9.15. Our social role-systems relate to the past, yet are stimulated in

Subphases in Authority Phase of Development	Survivor Roles That Are Triggered	Role-System Outputs That Are Modified
Flight	Social roles	Ambiguity, contradiction, redundancy, stereotyped subgrouping
	Explainer role	Explaining
	Identified patient	Posture, verbal pattern of identified patient
	Helper	Making suggestions to others
	Compliant	Going along
Transition to Fight	Complainer roles	Complaining rather than proposing
	Scapegoat	Bringing in differences that are "too-different"
	Scapegoater	Blaming, criticizing, targeting
	Dominant	Over-talking, interrupting, lengthy inputs
	Submissive	Head ducked, "apparently" going along
	Sadistic	Yes, but; opposing
	Masochistic	Blaming oneself when angry
	Defiant roles	No
Roles and Role Locks	One-up, one-down	Head raised, looking down on others or slumping and keeping eyes down
	Dominant/submissive roles	Bossy/acquiescent and yielding
Crisis of Hatred	Paranoid roles	Suspicious, quietly or challenging
	Defiant roles	Fighting against

Figure 9.15

the present by the whole system subphase dynamics and they function to maintain the subphase. Or as Yvonne described it many years earlier:

> Understanding projective identification as a function of group [system] dynamics allows the therapist to observe how the group role serves as the container for the group of those dynamics that are upsetting the group [system] equilibrium. Conceptually, understanding lies in recognizing the isomorphy between member roles (individual system) and group roles (group-as-a-whole system). Thus, group roles serve an equilibrating function that maintains the viability of the group by balancing forces that might otherwise disrupt it, even though, as in this group, the very mechanisms that keep the group equilibrium also fixate it and preclude further development.
>
> (Agazarian, 1987, p. 210)

Working with our role-systems map has deepened our appreciation for how modifying the restraining forces in phase-related role-system outputs impacts both the phase and the role-system itself. We have also learned how critically important it is to do this work in resonance with the inner-person, not in reactivity. Otherwise, the communication will not cross the boundary and will actually stimulate a more closed role, as we described doing in Chapter 3. When done in reactivity, the leader and member will be containing a role lock that maintains the system's phase. This is the way in which our person-as-a-system and role-systems maps have been so essential. They have enabled us to recognize how easily a survivor role activation in the leader can become a role lock iteration of the phase conflicts.

We have applied this in our SCT training for therapists where we emphasize the importance of learning to recognize and modify our own phase-related survivor roles so that we can listen to the conflicts of the inner-person on behalf of the system-as-a-whole rather than reenacting the repetition. On the other hand, when the repetition is reenacted and then recognized and explored, it can be undone most easily and usefully in the role lock phase.

Role-systems in the intimacy phase are affiliative/attachment roles

As the system transitions from its crisis of hatred with the leader, it transforms into the intimacy phase, where the relevant role-systems are the affiliative/attachment roles. We all develop these early in our lives with our caregivers and they are our past adaptations to our conflicts around separation/individuation.

Working with role-system outputs in therapy in the intimacy phase

The implicit intimacy phase goals are to either (1) idealize, a past adaptation that avoided separation and common for those of us who never separated, or (2) stay alienated from oneself and others, common in those of us who prematurely individuated (see Figure 9.16). These implicit goals are enacted in our past adaptive affiliative/attachment role-systems that maintain the past relationship to one's care-givers and repeat and relive it in the present. Once again, these repetitions maintain what we know, at the expense of opening to the unknown present. Patients often seek therapy when these role-systems are repeated in failed relationships and despair. In therapy, the intimacy work is with the early solutions as they are expressed in the here-and-now: this work is done by developing a functioning inter-person system (e.g., researcher, observer, subgrouping role) so that there is a context for the inner-person system development as the subgroups explore the phase-relevant roles.

Here too, the role-systems map is invaluable in guiding, identifying and modifying the role-system outputs. Again, our new understanding has proved vital in recognizing that when the differences that an intervention introduces can be integrated, the role-system itself can begin a process of development and ultimately transformation.

Intimacy	Survivor Role-Systems Related to Affiliative/Attachment Role-Systems	Role-System Outputs That Are Modified
Enchantment	Can't be close enough	Always agreeing, always seeing similarities
	Idealizing	Blind trust, not able to see differences
	Blind dependent	
Disenchantment	Alienated independent	Always seeing differences
	Self-alienated	Contempt and despair, blind mistrust of self and others, not able to see similarities

Figure 9.16

The collaborative phase in work teams and organizations

In organizations, it is in our collaborations with others that the affiliative/attachment roles impact our work (see Figure 9.17). As we discussed earlier, the focus on collaboration here is essential so that the language reflects the overarching context of organizations with their role, goal and context, quite different from the therapy context. Interestingly, the phase work in each context will be both similar and different. It is similar in that the phase is fueled by the same implicit goals and phase conflicts, yet the work is different in that the overarching system's context and goal are different. That is, in therapy, SCT works to develop the inter-person resources that are then inputs to the inner-person development. In organizations, the work is to develop the inter-person resources (fueled by the inner-person energy) that are then inputs to meet the whole system goal. This is of course an artificial discrimination, as when the inter-person system develops, it will impact up and down the hierarchy, yet the reality contexts have differential goals that support system development at different levels. The work with teams in this phase is to develop inter-person system capacity to collaborate towards common goals that support the goal of the context by weakening the role-system outputs that are restraining forces to the role, goal and context of the team.

Collaboration	Survivor Roles	Role-System Outputs That Are Modified
Emphasizing climate and maintenance	Resist autonomy	Focus on friendship/affiliation at expense of work goals
Focus on task over team	Go it alone role and ignoring the context and any similarities	Interrupting, building without reflecting Competing rather than working together
	Alienated independent role	Resist collaboration Always bringing a difference
	Avoidant role	Always working alone

Figure 9.17

In summary

We have summarized the SCT phases of system development and the application of SCT's phase model to clinical and training contexts as well as organizational and team development. We have also introduced our work in integrating our new role-systems map with our phase model. In SCT work, the phase context triggers the role-systems in the role-system hierarchy and is the context for the work that can be done. In closing this chapter, we cannot emphasize enough the importance in systems-centered work, whether the context is therapy or training or team development, of an in-depth understanding of the phases of system development and a capacity to diagnose the phase by identifying the implicit and explicit system output that enables identifying the role-systems and their goals. This recognition enables SCT practitioners to work in attunement with the resources of the phase context.

Note

1 Search of the terms "stages of group development" and "phases of group development" on July 5, 2019, resulted in a total of 2,555 articles.

References

Agazarian, Y. M. (1986). Application of Lewin's life space concept to the individual and group-as-a-whole systems in group psychotherapy. In E. Stivers & S. Wheelan (Eds.), *The Lewin legacy* (pp. 101–112). New York, NY: Springer-Verlag.

Agazarian, Y. M. (1987). The difficult patient, the difficult group: In Symposium: A discussion of the videotapes of a difficult group. *GROUP: The Journal of the Eastern Group Psychotherapy Society, 11*(4), 205–216. doi:10.1007/BF01459385

Agazarian, Y. M. (1999). Phases of development in the systems-centered group. *Small Group Research, 30*(1), 82–107. doi:10.1177/104649649903000105

Agazarian, Y. M., & Gantt, S. P. (2000). *Autobiography of a theory: Developing a theory of living human systems and its systems-centered practice.* London, UK: Jessica Kingsley.

Agazarian, Y. M., & Gantt, S. P. (2003). Phases of group development: Systems-centered hypotheses and their implications for research and practice. *Group Dynamics: Theory, Research and Practice, 7*(3), 238–252. doi:10.1037/1089-2699.7.3.238

Agazarian, Y. M., & Philibossian, B. (1998). A theory of living human systems as an approach to leadership of the future with examples of how it works. In E. Klein, F. Gabelnick, & P. Herr (Eds.), *The psychodynamics of leadership* (pp. 127–160). Madison, CT: Psychosocial Press.

Bennis, W. G., & Shepard, H. A. (1956). A theory of group development. *Human Relations, 9*(4), 415–437. doi:10.1177/001872675600900403

Brabender, V., & Fallon, A. (2009). *Group development in practice: Guidance for clinicians and researchers on stages and dynamics of change.* Washington, DC: American Psychological Association.

Gantt, S. P. (2005). Functional role-taking in organizations and work groups. *Group Psychologist (APA Division 49 Newsletter), 15*(5), 15.

Gantt, S. P. (2013). Applying systems-centered theory (SCT) and methods in organizational contexts: Putting SCT to work. *International Journal of Group Psychotherapy, 63*(2), 234–258. doi:10.1521/ijgp.2013.63.2.234

Gantt, S. P., & Agazarian, Y. M. (2004). Systems-centered emotional intelligence: Beyond individual systems to organizational systems. *Organizational Analysis, 12*(2), 147–169. doi:10.1108/eb028990

Gantt, S. P., & Agazarian, Y. M. (Eds.). (2005). *SCT in action: Applying the systems-centered approach in organizations.* Lincoln, NE: iUniverse. Reprint (2006). London, UK: Karnac Books.

Gantt, S. P., & Agazarian, Y. M. (2007). Phases of system development in organizational work groups: The systems-centered approach for intervening in context. *Organisational & Social Dynamics, 7*(2), 253–291.

Solomon-Gillis, C., & Trey, B. (1997). Applying systems-centered theory (SCT) to organizational consulting. *SCT Journal: Systems-Centered Theory and Practice, 2*, 39–42.

Wheelan, S., Burchill, C., & Tilin, F. (2003). The link between teamwork and patient outcomes in intensive care units. *American Journal of Critical Care, 12*(6), 527–534.

Wheelan, S., & Kesselring, J. (2005). The link between faculty group development and the performance of elementary students on standardized tests. *The Journal of Educational Research, 98*, 323–330.

Wheelan, S., & Lisk, A. (2000). Cohort group effectiveness and the educational achievement of adult undergraduate students. *Small Group Research, 31*(6), 724–738.

Wheelan, S., Murphy, D., Tsumura, E., & Fried Kline, S. (1998). Member perceptions of internal group dynamics and productivity. *Small Group Research, 29*(3), 371–393.

Wheelan, S., & Tilin, F. (1999). The relationship between faculty group effectiveness and school productivity. *Small Group Research, 30*(1), 59–81.

Epilogue

For those of you who made it this far, thank you for taking this journey with us. We have certainly developed as we thought, intuited, explored and wrote this book together. We hope you take with you the images and words that have resonated for you. We wish you curiosity as you discover how you might change as the images and words settle and integrate in you. And just as importantly, leave behind any images or words that don't resonate. Good-bye for now.

Appendix

SCT Theory Chart
SCT Phases of Development Chart
SCT Publications List

A THEORY OF LIVING HUMAN SYSTEMS

*A theory of living human systems defines a hierarchy of isomorphic systems:
energy-organizing, goal-directing and self-correcting*

THEORETICAL DEFINITIONS

HIERARCHY	ISOMORPHY		
Systems come in threes. Every system exists in the context of the system above & is the context for the system below.	Systems are similar in structure & function & different in different contexts. There is an interdependent relationship between the dynamics of structure, function & energy at all levels of the systems hierarchy.		
Context Systems-centered® contexts define a recursive triad of isomorphic systems in a defined hierarchy.	**Structure** Systems-centered structure defines boundaries in space, time & reality that are potentially permeable to energy/information.	**Energy** Systems-centered flow of energy/information is defined as a force field of vectors approaching or avoiding system goals.	**Function** Systems-centered function is to survive, develop & transform by discriminating & integrating differences & similarities.

SYSTEMS-CENTERED METHODS

Contextualizing: Activating the researcher role to perceive the isomorphy in the systems-centered hierarchy.	**Boundarying:** organizing system boundaries.	**Vectoring:** directing energy/information flow.	**Subgrouping:** correcting energy/information flow.
System-as-a-whole roles: Set norms & survive, develop & transform within the context of the defined hierarchy.	Survival: managing the permeability of system boundaries (in the hierarchy of systems) by reducing noise in the communications within & between all systems & subsystems.	Development: directing energy/information towards the primary goals of survival, development & transformation as well as the goals of the context.	Transformation: containing, discriminating & integrating differences in the apparently similar & similarities in the apparently different at all system levels.
Member system roles: Direct energy into subsystems. Discriminate & integrate information.			
Person system-as-a-whole: Source of primary energy/information flow.			

SYSTEMS-CENTERED TECHNIQUES

Eliciting the SCT® group requires activating the exploratory drive & contextualizing to establish the person, member, subgroup & group-as-a-whole system roles.	SCT techniques weaken the restraining forces to the flow of energy/information in the communications across the boundaries of the system hierarchy.	The "fork-in-the-road" techniques identify the choice between the restraining forces & the developmental driving forces.	The SCT conflict resolution technique of Functional Subgrouping enables containing, exploring & integrating differences instead of stereotyping or scapegoating them.

MAPS & INSTRUMENTS FOR DATA COLLECTION

Observations of the relationship between contextualizing, boundarying, vectoring & subgrouping interventions & role functions in crossing system boundaries.	**Past, Present & Future Reality/Irreality Map** **Phases of System Development Map** **SAVI®: System for Analyzing Verbal Interaction**	**The Force Field** **Hierarchy of Defense Modification Map**	**Functional Subgrouping Questionnaire (FSQ-2)**
Role, Goal & Context Map **Person-as-a-System Map** **Role-Systems Map**			

SCT® MODIFICATIONS OF RESTRAINING FORCES TO GROUP DEVELOPMENT

The chart below displays the forces that restrain the spontaneous drive towards system development. Column one displays the core conflict in each phase of system development. Column two displays the specific restraining forces that impede development of the individual system. Column three displays the symptoms generated by the conflicts that are modified when the restraining forces are reduced.

PHASE ONE OF GROUP DEVELOPMENT: AUTHORITY

FLIGHT SUBPHASE Impulse to contain dependency in the identified patient.	**SOCIAL DEFENSES** Stereotypic social communication.	Inauthenticity.
	THE TRIAD OF SYMPTOMATIC DEFENSES 1. Anxiety-provoking thoughts, ruminations and worrying that divert attention from reality-testing.	Anxiety.
	2. Tension-generating stress-related psychosomatic defenses which avoid the experience of emotion.	
TRANSITIONAL SUBPHASE BETWEEN FLIGHT AND FIGHT Impulse to target differences.	3. Defending against the retaliatory impulse by constricting it in depression or discharging it in hostile acting out.	Masochistic depression. Sadistic & hostile acting out.
FIGHT SUBPHASE Impulse to discharge hostility through scapegoating.	**ROLE LOCK DEFENSES** (interdependence of roles) Creating one-up/one-down role relationships like identified patient & helper; scapegoat & scapegoater; defiant & compliant.	Reciprocal maladaptive role pairing & role induction.
TRANSITIONAL SUBPHASE BETWEEN AUTHORITY AND INTIMACY Crisis of hatred, impulse to target authority.	**RESISTANCE TO CHANGE DEFENSES** 1. Externalizing conflicts onto those in authority: defensive stubbornness & suspicion from the righteous & complaining position.	Blaming authority for all problems.
	2. Disowning authority: defensive stubbornness & suspicion of self that blames personal incompetence.	Blaming self for all problems.

PHASE TWO OF GROUP DEVELOPMENT: INTIMACY (creating interdependence in relationships)

ENCHANTMENT AND HOPE SUBPHASE Impulses to idealize the group and create a cult.	**DEFENSES AGAINST SEPARATION** Enchantment, idealization, blind trust of others, merging & love addiction as defenses against differences.	Dependency at the expense of interdependence & exploitability.
DISENCHANTMENT AND DESPAIR SUBPHASE Impulses to alienate self in existential despair.	**DEFENSES AGAINST INDIVIDUATION** Disenchantment & blind mistrust of self, others & groups. Alienation, contempt & despair as a defense against similarities.	Independence at the expense of functional dependency & interdependence.

PHASE THREE OF GROUP DEVELOPMENT: INTERDEPENDENT (see here) LOVE, WORK & PLAY

ONGOING PHASES OF WORK IN THE EXPERIENCED GROUP Failures in response to the role, goal and context.	**DEFENSES AGAINST KNOWLEDGE** Defenses against inner reality & comprehensive & apprehensive knowledge.	Impairment of decision making & implementation abilities. Loss of common sense & humor.
	DEFENSES AGAINST COMMON SENSE Defenses against outer reality & reality-testing.	Self-centeredness at the expense of both self & the environment.

Developed by Yvonne M. Agazarian (2008).

© 2020 Systems-Centered Training & Research Institute, Inc.

SCT® and Systems-Centered® are registered trademarks of the Systems-Centered Training and Research Institute, Inc., a non-profit organization.

SCT publications

Agazarian, Y. M. (1982). Role as a bridge construct in understanding the relationship between the individual and the group. In M. Pines & L. Rafaelson (Eds.), *The individual and the group, boundaries and interrelations: Vol. I, theory* (pp. 181–192). New York, NY: Plenum Press.

Agazarian, Y. M. (1983a). Some advantages of applying multi-dimensional thinking to the teaching, practice and outcomes of group psychotherapy. *International Journal of Group Psychotherapy, 33*(2), 243–247. doi:10.1080/00207284.1983.11490871

Agazarian, Y. M. (1983b). Theory of invisible group applied to individual and group-as-a-whole interpretations. *GROUP: The Journal of the Eastern Group Psychotherapy Society, 7*(2), 27–37.

Agazarian, Y. M. (1986). Application of Lewin's life space concept to the individual and group-as-a-whole systems in group psychotherapy. In E. Stivers & S. Wheelan (Eds.), *The Lewin legacy* (pp. 101–112). New York, NY: Springer-Verlag.

Agazarian, Y. M. (1987). The difficult patient, the difficult group: In Symposium: A discussion of the videotapes of a difficult group. *GROUP: The Journal of the Eastern Group Psychotherapy Society, 11*(4), 205–216. doi:10.1007/BF01459385

Agazarian, Y. M. (1989a). Group-as-a-whole systems theory and practice. *GROUP: The Journal of the Eastern Group Psychotherapy Society, 13*(3–4), 131–155.

Agazarian, Y. M. (1989b). The invisible group: An integrational theory of group-as-a-whole: The 12th Annual Foulkes Memorial Lecture. *Group Analysis: The Journal of the Group Analytic Society, 22*(4), 74–96. doi:10.1177/0533316489224001

Agazarian, Y. M. (1991). Systems theory and group psychotherapy: From there-and-then to here-and-now. *The International Forum of Group Psychotherapy, 1*(3).

Agazarian, Y. M. (1992a). Contemporary theories of group psychotherapy: A systems approach to the group-as-a-whole. *International Journal of Group Psychotherapy, 42*(3), 177–203. doi:10.1080/00207284.1992.11490685

Agazarian, Y. M. (1992b). Friends Series I: System-centered theory & practice: In Y. M. Agazarian & SCTRI (Eds.), *Systems-centered theory and practice: The contribution of Yvonne Agazarian* (pp. 1–45). Livermore, CA: WingSpan Press. Reprint (2011). London, UK: Karnac Books.

Agazarian, Y. M. (1993). Reframing the group-as-a-whole. In T. Hugg, N. Carson, & R. Lipgar (Eds.), *Changing group relations: Proceedings of the ninth scientific meeting of the A.K. Rice Institute* (pp. 165–187). Juniper, FL: A.K. Rice Institute.

Agazarian, Y. M. (1994). The phases of group development and the systems-centred group. In M. Pines & V. Schermer (Eds.), *Ring of fire: Primitive object relations and affect in group psychotherapy* (pp. 36–85). London, UK: Routledge, Chapman & Hall.

Agazarian, Y. M. (1996a). Systems-centered therapy applied to short-term group and individual psychotherapy. *SCT Journal: Systems-Centered Theory and Practice, 1*, 23–34.

Agazarian, Y. M. (1996b). An up-to-date guide to the theory, constructs and hypotheses of a theory of living human systems and its systems-centered practice. *SCT Journal: Systems-Centered Theory and Practice, 1*, 3–12.

Agazarian, Y. M. (1997a). Glossary of SCT terms. *SCT Journal: Systems-Centered Theory and Practice, 2*, 3–10.

Agazarian, Y. M. (1997b). Systems-centered therapy. In H. G. Rosenthal (Ed.), *Favorite counseling and therapy techniques* (pp. 29–36). Washington, DC: Accelerated Development.

Agazarian, Y. M. (1997c). *Systems-centered therapy for groups.* New York, NY: Guilford. Reprinted in paperback (2004). London, UK: Karnac Books.

Agazarian, Y. M. (1999a). Phases of development in the systems-centered group. *Small Group Research, 30*(1), 82–107. doi:10.1177/104649649903000105

Agazarian, Y. M. (1999b). Systems-centered therapy. In J. Donigian & D. Hulse-Killacky (Eds.), *Critical incidents in group therapy.* Belmont, CA: Wadsworth.

Agazarian, Y. M. (1999c). Systems-centered supervision. *International Journal of Group Psychotherapy, 49*(2), 215–236. doi:10.1080/00207284.1999.11491582

Agazarian, Y. M. (2001). *A systems-centered approach to inpatient group psychotherapy.* London, UK and Philadelphia, PA: Jessica Kingsley.

Agazarian, Y. M. (2002). A systems-centered approach to individual and group psychotherapy. In L. Vandecreek & T. Jackson (Eds.), *Innovations in clinical practice: A source book* (Vol. 20, pp. 223–240). Sarasota, FL: Professional Resource Press.

Agazarian, Y. M. (2006). *Systems-centered practice: Selected papers on group psychotherapy.* London, UK: Karnac Books.

Agazarian, Y. M. (2010). *Systems-centered theory and practice: The contribution of Yvonne Agazarian* (SCTRI, Ed.). Livermore, CA: WingSpan Press. Reprint (2011). London, UK: Karnac Books.

Agazarian, Y. M. (2012a). Preface. In R. Lenn & K. Stefano (Eds.), *Small, large and median groups: The work of Patrick de Maré* (pp. xix–xxiv). London, UK: Karnac Books.

Agazarian, Y. M. (2012b). Systems-centered group psychotherapy: Putting theory into practice. *International Journal of Group Psychotherapy, 62*(2), 171–195. doi:10.1521/ijgp.2012.62.2.171

Agazarian, Y. M. (2012c). Systems-centered group psychotherapy: A theory of living human systems and its systems-centered practice. *GROUP: The Journal of the Eastern Group Psychotherapy Society, 36*(1), 19–36.

Agazarian, Y. M. (2016). Contrasting interpersonal and systems-centered approaches using two observation systems to analyze the communication patterns in two videotapes of the interpersonal approach to group psychotherapy. *GROUP: The Journal of the Eastern Group Psychotherapy Society, 40*(1), 71–88. doi:10.13186/group.40.1.0071

Agazarian, Y. M., & Byram, C. (2009). First build the system: The systems-centered approach to combined psychotherapy. *GROUP: The Journal of the Eastern Group Psychotherapy Society, 33*(2), 129–148.

Agazarian, Y. M., & Carter, F. (1993). The large group and systems-centered theory. *GROUP: The Journal of the Eastern Group Psychotherapy Society, 17*(4), 210–234.

Agazarian, Y. M., & Gantt, S. P. (2000). *Autobiography of a theory: Developing a theory of living human systems and its systems-centered practice.* London, UK: Jessica Kingsley.

Agazarian, Y. M., & Gantt, S. P. (2003). Phases of group development: Systems-centered hypotheses and their implications for research and practice. *Group Dynamics: Theory, Research and Practice, 7*(3), 238–252. doi:10.1037/1089-2699.7.3.238

Agazarian, Y. M., & Gantt, S. P. (2005a). The systems-centered approach to the group-as-a-whole. *GROUP: The Journal of the Eastern Group Psychotherapy Society, 29*(1), 163–186.

Agazarian, Y. M., & Gantt, S. P. (2005b). The systems perspective. In S. Wheelan (Ed.), *Handbook of group research and practice* (pp. 187–200). Thousand Oaks, CA: Sage Publications.

Agazarian, Y. M., & Gantt, S. P. (2014). Systems-centered training with couples: Building marriages that work. *Systemic Thinking & Psychotherapy, 5.*

Agazarian, Y. M., & Janoff, S. (1993). Systems theory and small groups. In I. Kaplan & B. Sadock (Eds.), *Comprehensive textbook of group psychotherapy* (3rd ed., pp. 33–44). Baltimore, MD: Williams & Wilkins, Division of Waverly.

Agazarian, Y. M., & Peters, R. (1981). *The visible and invisible group*. London, UK: Routledge & Kegan Paul. Reprinted in paperback (1987). London, UK: Karnac Books.

Agazarian, Y. M., & Philibossian, B. (1998). A theory of living human systems as an approach to leadership of the future with examples of how it works. In E. Klein, F. Gabelnick, & P. Herr (Eds.), *The psychodynamics of leadership* (pp. 127–160). Madison, CT: Psychosocial Press.

Åkerlund, M. (2017). Leadership: A team process developed through context awareness. *Scandinavian Journal of Organizational Psychology, 9*(2), 6–18.

Armington, R. (2012). Exploring the convergence of systems-centered therapy's functional subgrouping and the principles of interpersonal neurobiology. *Journal of Interpersonal Neurobiology Studies, 1,* 51–55.

Armington, R., & Cassano, S. M. (1996). The challenge of the member role in group problem solving. *SCT Journal: Systems-Centered Theory and Practice, 1,* 41–43.

Bateson, G. (1972). *Steps to an ecology of mind*. New York, NY: Ballantine Books.

Carter, F. (1996). Working with a large group in crisis: A systems-centered perspective. *SCT Journal: Systems-Centered Theory and Practice, 1,* 45–52.

Carter, F. (2000). Relationships as a function of context. In U. McCluskey & C. Hooper (Eds.), *Psychodynamic perspectives on abuse: The cost of fear*. London, UK and Philadelphia, PA: Jessica Kingsley.

Davis, R. (2013). Creating the conditions for all voices to be heard: Strategies for working with differences. *E-O&P Journal of the Association for Management Education and Development, 20*(1), 23–29.

Davis, R. (2014). Working across organisational boundaries: Shifting from complaining and blaming to problem-solving. *E-O&P Journal of the Association for Management Education and Development, 21*(3), 22–37.

Farrier, A., Davis, R., Froggett, L., & Poursanidou, K. (2010). "Shotgun partnership": A systems-centered case study analysis. *Journal of Place Management and Development, 3*(2), 136–148. doi:10.1108/17538331011062685

Forsmark, J. (2017). *Leading and teaching whitewater kayaking: Efficient outdoor leadership viewed from a theory of human living systems* (Master's thesis). Linköping University, Linköping, Sweden.

Ganley, R. (1997). Psychological and psycho-educational evaluations: Increasing the permeability of the reality-irreality and person-self boundaries. *SCT Journal: Systems-Centered Theory and Practice, 2,* 34–38.

Gantt, S. P. (1996). Defense analysis: Linking SCT theory and practice: Cognitive defenses. *SCT Journal: Systems-Centered Theory and Practice, 1,* 35–40.

Gantt, S. P. (1997). Similarities and differences. *SCT Journal: Systems-Centered Theory and Practice, 2,* 23–30.

Gantt, S. P. (2005). Functional role-taking in organizations and work groups. *Group Psychologist (APA Division 49 Newsletter), 15*(5), 15.

Gantt, S. P. (2009). The clinical pastoral circle: Using systems-centered methods to develop a clinical pastoral team. In C. F. Garlid, A. A. Zollfrank, & G. Fitchett (Eds.), *Expanding the circle: Essays in honor of Joan Hemenway* (pp. 109–136). Decatur, GA: Journal of Pastoral Care Publications.

Gantt, S. P. (2011). Functional subgrouping and the systems-centered approach to group therapy. In J. Kleinberg (Ed.), *The Wiley-Blackwell handbook of group psychotherapy* (pp. 113–138). Oxford, UK: Wiley.

Gantt, S. P. (2013). Applying systems-centered theory (SCT) and methods in organizational contexts: Putting SCT to work. *International Journal of Group Psychotherapy, 63*(2), 234–258. doi:10.1521/ijgp.2013.63.2.234

Gantt, S. P. (2015). Systems-centered group therapy. In E. S. Neukrug (Ed.), *Encyclopedia of theory in counseling and psychotherapy* (pp. 991–996). Thousand Oaks, CA: Sage Publications.

Gantt, S. P. (2018a). Developing groups that change our minds and transform our brains: Systems-centered's functional subgrouping, its impact on our neurobiology, and its role in each phase of group development. *Psychoanalytic Inquiry: Today's Bridge between Psychoanalysis and the Group World [Special Issue], 38*(4), 270–284. doi:10.1080/07351690.2018.1444851

Gantt, S. P. (2018b). In memoriam. Yvonne Agazarian. Group Circle, Winter.

Gantt, S. P. (2018c). In memory of Yvonne Agazarian, 1929–2017. *International Journal of Group Psychotherapy, 68*(2), 279–289. doi:10.1080/00207284.2017.1416792

Gantt, S. P. (2019a). Implications of neuroscience for group psychotherapy. In F. J. Kaklauskas & L. R. Greene (Eds.), *Core principles of group psychotherapy: An integrated theory, research, and practice training manual* (pp. 156–170). New York, NY: Routledge.

Gantt, S. P. (2019b). Yvonne M. Agazarian (1929–2017). *American Psychologist, 74*(2), 259. doi:10.1037/amp0000332

Gantt, S. P. (in press). Systems-centered theory (SCT) into group practice: Beyond surviving ruptures to repairing and thriving [special issue]. *International Journal of Group Psychotherapy*.

Gantt, S. P., & Adams, J. M. (2010). Systems-centered training for therapists: Beyond stereotyping to integrating diversities into the change process. *Women & Therapy, 33*(1), 101–120. doi:10.1080/02703140903404812

Gantt, S. P., & Agazarian, Y. M. (2004). Systems-centered emotional intelligence: Beyond individual systems to organizational systems. *Organizational Analysis, 12*(2), 147–169. doi:10.1108/eb028990

Gantt, S. P., & Agazarian, Y. M. (Eds.). (2005). *SCT in action: Applying the systems-centered approach in organizations.* Lincoln, NE: iUniverse. Reprint (2006). London, UK: Karnac Books.

Gantt, S. P., & Agazarian, Y. M. (Eds.). (2006). *Systems-centered therapy: In clinical practice with individuals, families and groups.* Livermore, CA: WingSpan Press. Reprint (2011). London, UK: Karnac Books.

Gantt, S. P., & Agazarian, Y. M. (2007). Phases of system development in organizational work groups: The systems-centered approach for intervening in context. *Organisational & Social Dynamics, 7*(2), 253–291.

Gantt, S. P., & Agazarian, Y. M. (2010). Developing the group mind through functional subgrouping: Linking systems-centered training (SCT) and interpersonal neurobiology. *International Journal of Group Psychotherapy, 60*(4), 515–544. doi:10.1521/ijgp.2010.60.4.515

Gantt, S. P., & Agazarian, Y. M. (2011a). The group mind, systems-centred functional subgrouping, and interpersonal neurobiology. In E. Hopper & H. Weinberg (Eds.), *The social unconscious in persons, groups, and societies: Volume 1: Mainly theory* (pp. 99–123). London, UK: Karnac Books.

Gantt, S. P., & Agazarian, Y. M. (2011b). Highlights from ten years of a systems-centered large group: Work in progress. *Voices: The Art and Science of Psychotherapy*, *47*(1), 40–50.

Gantt, S. P., & Agazarian, Y. M. (2017). Systems-centered group therapy. *International Journal of Group Psychotherapy*, *67*(sup1), S60–S70. doi:10.1080/00207284.2016.1218768

Gantt, S. P., & Badenoch, B. (Eds.). (2013). *The interpersonal neurobiology of group psychotherapy and group process*. London, UK: Karnac Books.

Gantt, S. P., & Badenoch, B. (2020). Systems-centered group psychotherapy: Developing a group mind that supports right brain function and right-left-right hemispheric integration. In R. Tweedy (Ed.), *The divided therapist: Hemispheric difference and contemporary psychotherapy*. London, UK: Routledge.

Gantt, S. P., & Cox, P. (Eds.). (2010). Introduction to the special issue: Neurobiology and building interpersonal systems: Groups, couples, and beyond [special issue]. *International Journal of Group Psychotherapy*, *60*(4), 455–460. doi:10.1521/ijgp.2010.60.4.455

Gantt, S. P., & Hopper, E. (2008a). Two perspectives on a trauma in a training group: The systems-centered approach and the theory of incohesion (part I). *Group Analysis*, *41*(1), 92–106. doi:10.1177/0533316408088416

Gantt, S. P., & Hopper, E. (2008b). Two perspectives on a trauma in a training group: The systems-centered approach and the theory of incohesion (part II). *Group Analysis*, *41*(2), 123–139. doi:10.1177/0533316408089879

Gantt, S. P., & Hopper, E. (2012). Two perspectives on a trauma in a training group: The systems-centered approach and the theory of incohesion. In E. Hopper (Ed.), *Trauma and organizations* (pp. 233–254). London, UK: Karnac Books.

Goldberg, S. (1997). Module 1 defense modification: Its application for short-term individual and group psychotherapy. *SCT Journal: Systems-Centered Theory and Practice*, *2*, 31–33.

Haddock, R. (2004). Drawing the isolate into the group flow: A commentary from a systems-centered therapy perspective. *Group Analysis*, *37*(1), 82–90.

Kahn, C. (1996). Evolution of group therapy from individual in the group to group-as-a-whole to group-as-a-system. *SCT Journal: Systems-Centered Theory and Practice*, *1*, 13–18.

Keane, W. M., & Weinstein, S. (1996). Rediscovering the self: Hard road to individuation. SCT in action with an Ashram community. *SCT Journal: Systems-Centered Theory and Practice*, *1*, 53–56.

Ladden, L. J., Gantt, S. P., Rude, S., & Agazarian, Y. M. (2007). Systems-centered therapy: A protocol for treating generalized anxiety disorder. *Journal of Contemporary Psychotherapy*, *37*(2), 61–70. doi:10.1007/s10879-006-9037-6

Maher, M. (2018). From group analytic to systems-centered consulting: A comparison of experience. *Journal of Social Work Practice*, *32*(4), 423–432. doi:10.1080/02650533.2018.1503163

McCluskey, U. (2002). The dynamics of attachment and systems-centered group psychotherapy. *Group Dynamics: Theory, Research and Practice*, *6*(2), 131–142.

McCluskey, U. (2005). *To be met as a person: The dynamics of attachment in professional encounters*. London, UK: Karnac Books.

McHenry, I. (1997). Integrating and transforming grief: A phenomenological account of a member's experience in a systems-centered group. *SCT Journal: Systems-Centered Theory and Practice*, *2*, 58–60.

Michael, T. A. (1997). Does that dream have a subgroup? The use of dreams in systems-centered theory. *SCT Journal: Systems-Centered Theory and Practice*, *2*, 18–22.

Murphy, V. (2007). *A longitudinal case study of effectiveness and efficiency in a systems-centered top management team* (Unpublished doctoral dissertation). Case Western Reserve University, Cleveland, OH.

O'Neill, R. M. (1996). Building an historical-empirical context for the systems-centered theory and practice. *SCT Journal: Systems-Centered Theory and Practice, 1*, 19–22.

O'Neill, R. M. (1997). Systems-centered theory and the trans-theoretical stages of change: Building a bridge of theory and data. *SCT Journal: Systems-Centered Theory and Practice, 2*, 11–17.

O'Neill, R. M. (2014). Systems-centered management: A brief review of theory, practice and research. *Review of Public Administration and Management, 2*(1). doi:10.4172/2315-7844.1000144

O'Neill, R. M., & Constantino, M. J. (2008). Systems-centered training groups' process and outcome: A comparison with AGPA institute groups. *International Journal of Group Psychotherapy, 58*(1), 77–102. doi:10.1521/ijgp.2008.58.1.77

O'Neill, R. M., Constantino, M. J., & Mogle, J. (2012). Does Agazarian's systems-centered functional subgrouping improve mood, learning and goal achievement?: A study in large groups. *Group Analysis, 45*, 375–390. doi:10.1177/0533316412448287

O'Neill, R. M., Gantt, S. P., Burlingame, G. M., Mogle, J., Johnson, J., & Silver, R. (2013). Developing the systems-centered functional subgrouping questionnaire-2. *Group Dynamics: Theory, Research, and Practice, 17*(4), 252–269. doi:10.1037/a0034925

O'Neill, R. M., & Mogle, J. (2015). Systems-centered functional subgrouping and large group outcome. *GROUP: The Journal of the Eastern Group Psychotherapy Society, 39*(4), 303–317. doi:10.13186/group.39.4.0303

O'Neill, R. M., Murphy, V., Mogle, J., MacKenzie, M. J., MacGregor, K. L., Pearson, M., & Parekh, M. (2013). Are systems-centered teams more collaborative, productive and creative? *Journal of Team Performance Management, 19*(3/4), 201–221. doi:10.1108/TPM-04-2012-0015

O'Neill, R. M., Reynolds, W., Culbertson, T., & Franklin, R. (2012). Systems-centered® training's functional subgrouping: A path to Koinonia in pastoral care. *Chaplaincy Today, 28*(1), 2–13. doi:10.1080/10999183.2012.10767443

O'Neill, R. M., Smyth, J. M., & MacKenzie, M. J. (2011). Systems-centered functional subgrouping links the member to the group dynamics and goals: How-to and a pilot study. *GROUP: The Journal of the Eastern Group Psychotherapy Society, 35*(2), 105–121.

Philibossian, B. (1996). Organizational application of the concept of functional subgrouping. *SCT Journal: Systems-Centered Theory and Practice, 1*, 62–64.

Robbins, M. R. (1996). Group therapy for body, mind and spirit: A systems-centered approach. *SCT Journal: Systems-Centered Theory and Practice, 1*, 57–61.

Robbins, M. R. (1997). Contacting the numinous and creative work at the edge of the unknown in a systems-centered therapy context. *SCT Journal: Systems-Centered Theory and Practice, 2*, 52–57.

Simon, A. (1993). Using SAVI for couples' therapy. *Journal of Family Psychotherapy, 4*, 39–62.

Simon, A. (1996). SAVI and individual SCT therapy. *SCT Journal: Systems-Centered Theory and Practice, 1*, 65–71.

Simon, A., & Agazarian, Y. M. (1967). *SAVI: Sequential analysis of verbal interaction.* Philadelphia, PA: Research for Better Schools.

Simon, A., & Agazarian, Y. M. (2000). SAVI: The system for analyzing verbal interaction. In A. P. Beck & C. M. Lewis (Eds.), *The process of group psychotherapy: Systems for analyzing change* (pp. 357–380). Washington, DC: American Psychological Association.

Solomon-Gillis, C., & Trey, B. (1997). Applying systems-centered theory (SCT) to organizational consulting. *SCT Journal: Systems-Centered Theory and Practice, 2*, 39–42.

Tschuschke, V. (1997). A summary of process-outcome relationships in a systems-centered group compared with the effects of other special interest groups (SIG groups) at the 1996 AGPA Institute. *SCT Journal: Systems-Centered Theory and Practice, 2*, 61–63.

Whitcomb, K., O'Neill, R. M., Burlingame, G. M., Mogle, J., Gantt, S. P., Cannon, J., & Rooney, T. (2018). Measuring how systems-centered® members connect with group dynamics: FSQ-2 construct validity. *International Journal of Group Psychotherapy, 68*(2), 163–183. doi:10.1080/00207284.2017.1381024

For other SCT resources, see www.systemscentered.com

Index

Note: Page numbers in *italic* indicate a figure on the corresponding page. Page numbers followed by 'n' indicate a note.